# A SMALL DOSE OF TOXICOLOGY

## The Health Effects of Common Chemicals

# A SMALL DOSE OF
# TOXICOLOGY

## The Health Effects of Common Chemicals

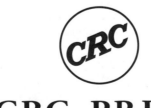

## Steven G. Gilbert, PhD, DABT

Director, Institute of Neurotoxicology
and Neurological Disorders
Seattle
USA

**CRC**

# CRC PRESS

Boca Raton   London   New York   Washington, D.C.

## Library of Congress Cataloging-in-Publication Data

Gilbert, Steven G., 1951-
    A small dose of toxicology / Steven G. Gilbert.
        p.   cm.
    Includes bibliographical references and index.
    ISBN 0-415-31168-3
    1. Toxicology—Popular works. I. Title.

RA1213 .G54 2003
615.9—dc21                                                                2003055232

**Visit the CRC Press Web site at www.crcpress.com**

# Contents

# Preface

Historically toxicology has focused on poisonous chemicals with death as the primary endpoint, but my interest in toxicology began when I realized that even small amounts of a chemical could irrevocably damage the brain of the developing child, resulting in a lifetime of harm. Knowing that a high level of exposure to a chemical can kill an animal, insect, plant or human is no longer as relevant as the knowledge that repeated exposure to chemicals at low levels can cause brain damage or cancer. The knowledge that children exposed to commonly used chemicals could be permanently affected for a lifetime seemed to me both profound and tragic. Thus, my initial interest and primary focus was on how chemicals affect the developing brain, particularly on the effects of exposure to lead and mercury.

During the 1960s and 1970s researchers and physicians documented that heavy metals, such as lead and mercury, could seriously harm the developing infant. While high levels of exposure resulted in death or obviously serious consequences, the harmful effects from low levels of exposure remained unexplored. The laboratory I worked in designed and performed studies that ultimately demonstrated that even very low levels of exposure to lead or mercury could harm the developing nervous system. The fundamental issue was not death, but quality of life and the consequences for the individual, particularly sensitive individuals such as children.

The results of our research were exciting, but immediately raised the issue of how to use this information to protect sensitive individuals, particularly children. The widespread use and environmental distribution of these agents meant that the health and well-being of the individual could be protected only by changes in government regulation. My perspective on toxicology had to broaden to include issues well outside the laboratory. At that time, lead was commonly used as a gasoline additive and mercury was common in many industrial applications, which resulted in widespread environmental distribution and subsequent human exposure. Convincing the various government and industry groups of the importance of drastically reducing environmental exposure was difficult because exposure did not appear to cause any overtly visible harm at low levels. Only the government could establish broad policies or regulation that could reduce individual exposure to these chemicals and thus protect sensitive individuals. While the government has an essential role to play, it is also clear that individuals need to understand the principles of toxicology involved in these issues.

Knowledge about the adverse effects of agents or toxicology influences many decisions that ultimately shape our lives and guide our society. Medical drugs undergo extensive testing to ensure efficacy and to understand possible toxic side effects. Much of the government-mandated testing of commercial agents came only after a clear example of toxicity. Following a near disastrous experience with DDT, pesticides now must undergo a battery of tests to evaluate both environmental effects as well as effects on people, although many of these tests still only evaluate the active ingredients. However, the inherent toxicity of pesticides causes undesirable health and environmental effects when they are inappropriately or excessively utilized, and in some cases even when used properly. Food additives, such as artificial sweeteners, are evaluated prior to use in the food supply to ensure that there are no long-term health effects for even the most sensitive individuals. Environmental contaminants, such as mercury, in the food supply result in restrictive local fishing rules as well as regulations on international fish stocks. National and international regulations are in place to reduce pollution in the air, water, and soil, but there is ongoing debate as to whether these regulations are adequate. These are but a few examples of how the science of toxicology influences our lives. Ultimately it is our individual understanding of the principles of toxicology and our willingness to become involved with the process that will have the greatest impact on our local and global environment.

The basic principles of toxicology can explain many things in our lives as well as enlighten our understanding of current and historical events. As we shall see, there are sound physiological reasons why the coffee, tea, and cola industries make money from caffeine. The lens of toxicology brings a different focus to historical events. For example, the toxicological properties of opium are the subplot to many a war over drugs. The opium wars between Great Britain and China resulted in Hong Kong being ceded to Great Britain. Today, drug wars continue in various forms around the world and have enormous consequences for countries and individuals. The daily news offers many current examples of the undesirable effects of agents and demonstrates the ongoing impact of the principles of toxicology.

One of the most basic principles of toxicology is that the amount of exposure, or dose, determines the beneficial and harmful effects of a substance. In toxicology this is commonly referred to as dose–response or "the dose makes the poison." Paracelsus (1493–1541) eloquently stated this concept as "All substances are poisons; there is none which is not a poison. The right dose differentiates a poison from a remedy". For example, drugs taken to control or cure cancer are often very toxic, and it is only the amount taken that separates the beneficial effects from outright death. While this principle is accurate, it leaves out the very important concept of individual sensitivity. The sensitivity of the individual must be considered when evaluating the potential harm of exposure to the agent. It is not particularly important to know how much lead it takes to kill a child; the critical issue is how much lead it takes to cause brain damage and harm that child's potential for a lifetime.

All life is born with a certain potential inscribed in its genes. Advances in molecular biology and genomic sciences are now letting us look directly at the coding of the gene. The toxicological sciences provide insight into how this genetic potential is damaged by its interaction with chemical or physical agents. Combining the knowledge gained through the toxicological and genomic sciences leads to a new definition of environmental health.

---

**Environmental Health**

Conditions that ensure that all living things have the best opportunity to reach and maintain their full genetic potential.

Steven G. Gilbert, 1999

---

To ensure the health and well-being of our children and all life we must protect the genetic potential of the individual. Even a low level of lead exposure during childhood may rob the child of its genetic potential. The concept of dose–response must be expanded to include the sensitive individual and protecting genetic potential.

With a little imagination, the principle of dose and response easily expands beyond the normal concepts of toxicology and poisons. We are constantly being dosed or exposed to all manners of things to which we respond. For example, you are getting a small dose of this book right now. What is your response? Will you read further or close the book? Most of you have already had a first dose of this book from a quick scan of the Contents or from flipping through the pages; from there the response was to read more.

I developed a very expansive view of toxicology in which the basic principles were applicable from the smallest to the most encompassing issues. The utility of using toxicology to demystify many current and historical issues developed gradually for me, while trying to teach students and other groups about toxicology. University lectures are often highly focused on very specific topics such as changes in the developing nervous system following lead exposure. But the real challenge lies in teaching the basic principles of toxicology to interested adults, high school, and even elementary school pupils. My early effort to share the explanatory powers of toxicology began when I joined the Master Home Environmentalist program. This group held classes to instruct homeowners and renters about how to reduce exposures to toxic substances in and around the home. The challenge was to make toxicology both interesting and relevant. Teaching in high school and elementary school classes further emphasized the importance of making toxicology relevant to our daily lives.

I soon discovered that most people already know a great deal about toxicology, even though they may not realize it. The ultimate purpose of this book is to bring this knowledge to light by putting a conceptual framework around our everyday knowledge of toxicology. This book is a tool to help people learn about toxicology so they can form their own opinions about the potential harm from any exposure and develop ways to reduce exposure. Knowing the underlying principles of toxicology allows for far more effective analysis of a problem or situation and thus more effective decision-making. This book is not a comprehensive survey of hazardous chemicals but uses everyday examples to illustrate the principles of toxicology. The field of toxicology has many textbooks addressing the finer points of chemistry, biology, and mechanisms of action but few that explain toxicology as part of our day-to-day issues of living. To facilitate learning or teaching this material, additional references and a *PowerPoint* presentation are available for each chapter at www.asmalldoseof.org or at http://www.crcpress.com/e_products/ (follow the links to downloads and then the catalog number TF1691).

I hope you find this book a useful tool for exploring toxicology, that it provides you with insight into your everyday choices, and that it adds to the foundation and power of your individual decision-making.

# Acknowledgments

The idea for this book germinated while preparing to teach a continuing education course on toxicology for the Department of Environmental and Occupational Health Sciences at the University of Washington. I wish to thank the staff in the Continuing Education program for the opportunity to develop some of this material as well as many of the instructors who gave lectures. In particular I want to thank Gerald van Belle, at that time Chair of the Department of Environmental Health, for introducing one of the continuing education programs as "A Small Dose of Toxicology". Parts of the first two chapters were originally developed for the Master Home Environmentalist (MHE) program as a section of their training manual. The MHE program trains volunteers to help people reduce hazardous exposure in their homes. This book is for the volunteers. Philip Dickey encouraged me to "get on with it." He provided a first draft of the chapter on home toxics, read all the chapters and provided many substantive and editorial comments. Finally, I want to thank Janice Camp for her ongoing support in all ways large and small.

# Chapter 1

# Toxicology and you

## Contents

- Everyday examples of toxicology
- Toxicological resources

Toxicology originally developed as the study of poisons and is now more formally described as the study of the adverse effects of chemical or physical agents on living organisms. During our lives, most of us begin to develop an intuitive sense of toxicology that guides many of our personal day-to-day decisions. This process can start first thing in the morning over a cup of coffee or tea or a can of cola. These common beverages contain caffeine, the most widely consumed stimulant in the world. Most consumers of caffeine are well aware of the benefits of this drug as well as the consequences of consuming too much. Through trial and error we have learned how to moderate our consumption of caffeine to avoid any undesirable effects. In regulating our consumption of caffeine we are applying the most basic principle of toxicology: dose–response. We apply this principle as we judge how much and what to eat or drink, or how much suntan lotion we should use before going to the beach. As we shall see in a future chapter, caffeine provides an excellent example of how we apply knowingly or unknowingly the principles of toxicology. Understanding how caffeine interacts with the body can even explain why the coffee and soft drink companies make so much money from this amazing drug. Looking at the world through the lens of toxicology provides a very interesting perspective on current, historical, and personal events.

The purpose of *A Small Dose of Toxicology* is to build upon our intuitive understanding of toxicology and make it the basis for the knowledgeable and comfortable application of the principles of toxicology. Placing some form and structure around what we already intuitively know about toxicology will allow more critical analysis of not only our immediate environment but many of the current events that shape our local and global society. Toxicological considerations shape directly or indirectly many decisions about our home, play, school, or work environments. As citizens in a democratic society, we must be able to meaningfully engage decision makers in industry, government, and the news media to influence the development of our local environment as well as society. This book is not about the thousands of commercial chemicals that are in use, but rather about the principles that guide decisions about their use and distribution. A little knowledge about toxicology will allow us to judge the potential effect on our lives better, ask insightful questions, and ultimately influence the decision makers.

Historically, toxicology was most often concerned with how much of a substance it took to kill you. Literature has some splendid examples of the awareness of naturally occurring poisons. The ancient Greeks were very knowledgeable about the properties of the hemlock plant, part of the parsley family, even though they did not know what specific chemical in it caused death. In 399 BC Socrates was condemned to die by hemlock after being charged with religious heresy and corrupting the morals of local youth. We now know that the active chemical is the alkaloid coniine, which when ingested causes paralysis, convulsions, and potentially death. More modern examples of the knowledge of poisons can be seen in the following from a well-known playwright, Shakespeare:

> Come bitter pilot, now at once run on
> The dashing rocks thy seasick weary bark!
> Here's to my love! O true apothecary!
> Thy drugs are quick. Thus with a kiss I die.
> From *Romeo and Juliet* – Act 5

Historical events can also be interpreted from the perspective of toxicology. For example, Great Britain acquired Hong Kong during the Opium War of 1839–42, which was really about the toxic and additive properties of this opium. Medical uses of opium included the treatment of diseases such as dysentery and cholera. Users soon found that smoking a mixture of tobacco and opium increased the absorption of opium, resulting in a more rapid onset of its effects. The Chinese government was trying to curb the smoking of opium because of its debilitating effects, which was at odds with the British desire to increase the opium trade. The sale of all narcotics including opium was made illegal in the United States in 1923. The popularity of drug use continues and governments are engaged in a variety of efforts to curb their use, including "drug wars" with neighboring countries.

Knowledge about the physiological and toxicological properties of drugs (legal or illegal) is important in developing sound public policy. Looking at historical and current events through the filter of toxicology (see below) provides a new perspective on the underlying issues. Life has many examples of toxicology, if one only thinks or sees in terms of a toxicologist.

## 1.1 Everyday examples of toxicology

Below are a few examples (Table 1.1); there are many more, and they occur every day in the news. Can you add to this list? What toxicology related or biology related issues have been in the news recently?

## Table 1.1 Everyday examples of toxicology

| What aspect of toxicology? | Comment |
| --- | --- |
| Thalidomide | Developed as a sedative in the early 1960s but found to cause a rare birth defect, phocomelia. In 1962 legislation was passed that new drugs must undergo sufficient animal and human testing prior to approval for use by the US FDA. |
| Hong Kong | (a) Many chickens and birds in Hong Kong were killed to stop the spread of a potentially deadly avian virus that could move to humans.<br>(b) Why was Hong Kong a British colony? This was in part due to the opium wars, when England and other countries wanted to promote the use of opium to the Chinese population. Consider the current US "war on drugs". |
| Princess Diana | At the time of death her driver may have had too much alcohol to drink. |
| Ambassador to Mexico | A number of years ago a former governor of Massachusetts (Weild) was denied the opportunity to become the ambassador to Mexico because US Senator Jesse Helms thought he was "soft on drugs". Yet this senator was from a key tobacco growing state and a major supporter of the tobacco industry (and hence nicotine). Who is soft on drugs? |
| $276 Billion | Money lost or spent due to the consumption of alcohol or drug abuse, car accidents, lost work, etc. . . . |
| $65 Billion | Money lost or spent due to tobacco related illnesses or disease. |
| Food | Our food supply is produced using, and is contaminated with, pesticides. Artificial sweeteners, flavors, and colors are used. Mercury contaminates some fish. |
| Noise | Loud noise can damage hearing and can cause an even greater effect in combination with certain drugs. |
| Dust | The dust in your home may contain many hazardous contaminants, e.g., lead or pesticides. Many of these can be brought into the home on shoes or by pets. Removing shoes can reduce contamination in the home. |
| 12,000 Children | Estimated number of children with fetal alcohol syndrome. |
| Coeur d'Alene, Silver Valley, ID | Town contaminated by lead. |
| Solar radiation (ultraviolet light) | Sunburn, cancer. |
| Arsenic | Found in drinking water, and old smelter and mining sites, causes skin disease and cancer. |

Toxicology, while formally considered a new science, has ancient roots and is closely linked to medicine. Toxicology's counterpart in medicine is pharmacology, the study of the beneficial and side effects of medicinal drugs. The adverse effects of drugs, often termed side effects, are really the toxicological or undesired aspects of the drug that one must endure along with the benefits. The basic principles of pharmacology and toxicology are very similar, with just a different emphasis on the outcome. For example, one can study both the pharmacological or beneficial aspects of caffeine and at the same time be looking at the undesired or toxicological aspects of too much caffeine. Caffeine at the right dose is commonly consumed for its stimulant effects on the nervous system, but too much produces equally recognizable and undesirable effects.

As knowledge of the effects of poisons grew so did the definition of toxicology. A more contemporary definition of toxicology is the study of the adverse (undesired or harmful) effects of chemical and physical agents on living organisms. While this definition may appear relatively simple there are important aspects worth exploring. "Adverse effects" can range from obvious ones like death, cancer, an injury such as an acid burn, or the undesired effects of too much caffeine. We quickly note these unpleasant effects and easily relate them to the consumption of or exposure to the agent. As our understanding of toxicology has increased, there has been a shift in focus to recognizing the unique sensitivity of individuals and to more subtle effects such as a decrease in learning and memory. Subtle damage to the nervous system, which can result in a decrease in intelligence, is more difficult to assess in an individual and to relate to exposure. To assess subtle changes it is often necessary to evaluate exposure and effect in a large group or population of people. Our increased awareness of the adverse effects of lead exposure on young children is an excellent example of the changing perspective on toxicology. It is not nearly as important to know how much lead will kill a child as it is to understand the sensitivity of the child's developing brain to even low levels of exposure to lead. Harming the learning and memory of a child results in a lifetime of undesirable effects and consequences for the individual and society.

The child pictured in Figure 1.1 working in a lead battery recycling factory in Bangladesh illustrates the global implications of toxicology. This child will suffer from the effects of lead poisoning for a lifetime and will not be able to reach his intellectual potential.

The second part of the definition of toxicology concerns "chemical or physical agents". Chemical agents can be either naturally occurring or manufactured. Hazardous naturally occurring agents produced by living organisms are called toxins while hazardous manufactured agents are called toxicants. Naturally occurring agents can be as benign and essential as water or as deadly as the venom of a coral snake. Plants, animals, and bacteria produce a range of chemical substances or toxins that usually aid in their survival or defense. Humans and even other animals have learned to use these agents to cure disease as well as poison other plants and animals. Several different plants produce caffeine, a bitter compound, most likely to protect them from insects. Digitalis, from foxglove, is used in treating heart disease. Bacteria, such as botulism or anthrax, produce toxins that can kill humans, but we take advantage of the yeast that produces alcohol. Our industrial society has learned to manufacture a wide range of chemicals designed for specific purposes.

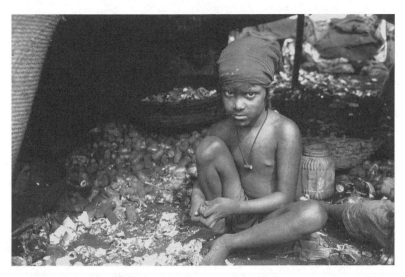

*Figure 1.1.* Child working in a lead battery recycling factory (with permission from Still Pictures/Peter Arnold Inc.).

Much of our food supply depends on the use of pesticides. Our households, schools and workplaces contain numerous chemicals that are potentially hazardous. The laptop computer essential for writing this book contains thousands of different chemicals. The manufacture of many of the items we depend upon and their subsequent disposal can create additional hazards. There are numerous examples around the world of contaminated areas that are potentially hazardous to animals, plants, and humans.

Physical agents represent a different set of challenges for a toxicologist and are often related to occupational health issues. Temperature and noise are the two most common physical agents that must be considered. In the past decade there has been a growing recognition of the harmful effects of loud noise on hearing and, even more important, a willingness to promote the use of hearing protectors. Changes in stream temperature can affect the ability of fish to live and reproduce. Excessive temperature in the work environment or from wearing protective clothing can decrease performance. Both noise and temperature can increase the stress in the environment and interact with other agents to produce a significant decline in performance. Some drugs can interact with noise to produce greater hearing loss. Sleep deprivation or jet lag can also have serious undesirable effects or just an annoying temporary loss of performance.

Toxicology has progressed along with the biological sciences to place a greater emphasis on understanding the mechanism of action of an agent, greater focus on the subtle responses of the organism, and recognition of the sensitivity of individuals. Thus toxicology has moved away from death as an endpoint to a focus on performance and quality of life. Exposure to hazardous vapor may result in impaired judgment or slowed reaction time, resulting in serious injury to the person responding to an emergency. The child exposed to alcohol during gestation may have permanent learning disabilities because of the sensitivity of the developing brain at that particular point. Recognition that the sensitivity of the individual depends on stage of development, age, or genetic makeup has become one of the most important principles of toxicology. This has modified the thinking and application of the principle of dose–response.

It is possible to take an even broader view of toxicology by defining it as the study of the response of a defined system to some event or exposure to an agent. The principles of toxicology are now applicable to vast systems such as consideration of global warming or the effects of logging on the rainforest. Increased atmospheric carbon dioxide is a toxic event which results in a response of global warming. What dose of logging can a rainforest sustain? The basic principles of toxicology are a framework for considering the small local events to large global events or entire biosystems, which moves us into ecological considerations. Application of the principles of toxicology to even very large events where there is an action or exposure or a reaction and a response results in a simplification that can lead to a unique perspective. However, this more ecological perspective on toxicology is not the subject of the book but is worth keeping in mind as one applies the principles of toxicology on a day-to-day basis.

An underlying theme behind this book is to place toxicology in the context of environmental health. How do you define environmental health? What environment are we considering – home, school, workplace, outdoors, indoors, the oceans, the air, or water? I define environmental health as "Conditions that ensure that all living things have the best opportunity to reach and maintain their full genetic potential". While this is a very broad approach to environmental health, its value can be best illustrated by looking at children. How do we ensure that our children can reach their "full genetic potential"? For example, children exposed to even very low levels of lead may have learning disabilities. These detrimental changes may affect the child for a lifetime. How do we as individuals and as a society work to ensure that children are not adversely affected by exposure to lead? This is a complex issue that goes well beyond toxicology, but knowing more about toxicology can help in making small decisions that can influence a child's future quality of life. The same is true of larger environmental issues. A *Small Dose of Toxicology* strives to apply the principles of toxicology to the broader goal of increasing the potential of all living things to have an opportunity to reach and maintain their full genetic inheritance. We will examine the effects of exposure to specific agents on living systems and emphasize changes in performance and function.

Ensuring environmental health is a complex interaction of the individual as well as society and ranges from the local to the global. Gold miners in the Amazon use mercury to extract the gold. As the mercury evaporates to reveal the gold, it harms the miners as they breathe it in, but mercury is also going into the atmosphere. The wind may take the mercury in the atmosphere far away but eventually it comes back to the ground, where it is modified by bacteria and taken up by fish. Government agencies must then regulate the amount of mercury acceptable in certain species of fish such as tuna and swordfish. Broken thermometers, fluorescent light bulbs, and a variety of consumer products release mercury into the environment. As a society, how much do we spend to curb the release or even the sale of mercury?

Pesticides are chemicals designed to kill unwanted plants, insects, and animals. While necessary in some situations, their widespread use has had unintended consequences. DDT, widely used to kill mosquitoes, is but one example. It was subsequently found to weaken bird shell eggs, causing serious declines in predatory birds. An interesting property of DDT and a number of related pesticides is that they can be stored in fat. As DDT moves up the food chain from smaller to larger animals more and more accumulates in the fat. During breast feeding, fat is mobilized and along with it the DDT, which appears in the breast milk consumed by the infant. These are two of the many examples that we must confront as we begin to appreciate the global implication of toxicology and environmental health and impacts on individuals.

State and national government agencies spend our tax dollars on environmental and toxicology issues. Both the US Food and Drug Administration (FDA) and the Environmental Protection Agency (EPA) were formed in an effort to protect the health and well-being of people and the environment. For both agencies, 1962 was a year to remember. A turning point in the regulation governing the FDA occurred in 1962 when it was determined that a new sleeping pill, thalidomide, was shown to cause birth defects. Infants in Europe and Australia were born with birth defects when pregnant women used thalidomide. Fortunately, Dr. Frances O. Kelsey, an FDA scientist, kept this drug off the American market despite the best efforts of industry to have the drug approved. Following this incident, regulation was passed that significantly strengthened the FDA's control over approval of new drugs. Also in 1962, Rachel Carson published her landmark book *Silent Spring*, which dramatically documented the impact of chemicals on the environment and raised concerns about the effect of pesticides on human health. In a delayed political response, the EPA was created in 1970 to administer a variety of laws to protect human health and the environment. The EPA is responsible for regulating the use of pesticides, industrial chemicals, hazardous waste, drinking water, air pollutants and other environmental hazards. These two agencies, as well as other federal and state agencies, spend a lot of money based on principles of toxicology.

The title of this book, *A Small Dose of Toxicology*, identifies a primary aim, which is to provide a small but useful introduction to toxicology. Many of the examples were selected to emphasize how toxicology fits into everyday events and life choices. Do we take one or two cups of coffee? What are the consequences of drinking alcohol or the consumption of other recreational drugs? Why are some individuals more sensitive than others? Was food cooked long enough to ensure that all bacteria are killed? My focus is on the practical application of toxicology in our day-to-day lives, but I want to keep a perspective on applying the principles of toxicology to bigger issues. I omitted some of the details on the chemistry and mechanisms of action knowing that this information is available from other sources. A list of references includes a number of excellent books that contain more specific information on the chemistry and mechanisms of action of both common and obscure toxic agents. It is said that toxicology can be learned in two easy lessons of only 10 years each (I think it may be three lessons now). This book is an introduction to the first 10 years.

Understanding the principles of toxicology can provide the power to discover new insights into decision-making. The principles of toxicology can then be applied to ever changing circumstances as we search for some understanding of the issues. The power is in having the knowledge to evaluate a new situation.

It is not the truth that makes you free. It is your possession of the power to discover the truth. Our dilemma is that we do not know how to provide that power.
Roger Lewontin, *New York Review of Books*, Jan 7, 1997

Each of us can benefit from discovering how and why our bodies interact with an agent as well as from understanding how various compounds impact the environment. Appreciating the impact of dose–response and individual susceptibility provides a basis upon which to take action to improve our own health and well-being and that of the environment. Knowing that an infant is more susceptible than an adult to an agent such as lead, because of their low weight and sensitivity of their developing nervous systems, can result in small but important actions that reduce the infant's exposure and thus improve the quality of life. This knowledge may also translate into changes in the workplace or by government agencies. Knowledge can provide the power to shape and influence environmental health.

The "Principles of toxicology" chapter provides an overview of the principles of toxicology while subsequent chapters explore specific topics in greater depth. The reader is encouraged to pick and choose specific areas of interest; toxicology is fun when explored out of curiosity. One unique feature of the book is that each chapter has a corresponding *PowerPoint* presentation. This presentation material was designed to aid the student or the teacher by providing a concise overview of the material in the chapter and, in some cases, provide information from a slightly different perspective. A teacher can use this material for classroom presentation or the student can use the presentation material as class notes or for review of the chapter material. As a teacher myself, I have always wondered how many times the same material has been reproduced to accommodate a lecture.

## 1.2 Toxicological resources

There is a large and ever-growing body of information on toxicology, particularly on the World Wide Web. Many national government, international organization and non-government agencies have excellent web sites with detailed information on the issues discussed in this book. I urge you to consult these sites for more in-depth information. Your local bookstore, particularly a large university bookstore or an ecologically oriented store, may have additional information. Unfortunately much of the in-depth medical or highly scientific information is not very accessible. There are also many non-governmental organizations that can provide additional information and a different perspective. Computer networks and local public and university libraries also contain a wealth of information. Teaching aids, including material directly related to this book, are also available on-line or from a variety of organizations.

Below is a list and brief description of a very few of the more detailed web sites and references. Each chapter has additional specific resources and references, while those below are more general in nature.

## 1.2.1 Teaching resources

■ Toxicology and You presentation material. Online. Available HTTP: <http://www.crcpress.com/e_products/> and follow the links to downloads and then the catalog number TF1691.
Web site contains presentation material related to this book for each chapter.

■ Center for Ecogenetics and Environmental Health, Department of Environmental and Occupational Health Sciences, University of Washington. Online. Available HTTP: <http://depts.washington.edu/ceeh/Outreach/outreach.html> (accessed: 1 April 2003).
K-12 teacher resources, Tox-In-A-Box, and other teacher and student aids.

■ Toxicology Tutorials – National Library of Medicine. Online. Available HTTP: <http://sis.nlm.nih.gov/Tox/ToxTutor.html> (accessed: 1 April 2003).
Site has three tutorial lessons on toxicology.

■ Toxicology Education Foundation (TEF). Online. Available HTTP: <http://www.toxicology.org/publicoutreach/tef/tef.html> (accessed: 2 April 2003).
TEF provides grants and resources for education in toxicology.

■ Society of Toxicology (SOT) – K-12 Resources. Online. Available HTTP: <http://www.toxicology.org/publicoutreach/k12resources/k-12educators.html> (accessed: 2 April 2003).
US national toxicology organization site has a variety of useful information and links to educational resources on toxicology and related biological sciences.

## 1.2.2 European, Asian, and international agencies

■ Organization For Economic Co-Operation And Development (OECD) – Chemical Safety. Online. Available HTTP: <http://www.oecd.org/> (accessed: 10 April 2003).
This OECD Site contains general information on environmental and chemical health and safety.

■ European Union – Public Health. Online. Available HTTP: <http://europa.eu.int/pol/health/index_en.htm> (accessed: 4 April 2003).
European Union has extensive health related information in many languages.

■ European Environment Agency. Online. Available HTTP: <http://www.eea.eu.int/> (accessed: 9 April 2003).
European Environment Agency has extensive environmental health related information in many languages.

■ The National Institute for Clinical Excellence (NICE). Available HTTP: <http://www.cdc.gov/niosh/ipcsneng/nengsyn.html> (accessed: 2 April 2003).
NICE was set up as a Special Health Authority for England and Wales and its role is to provide patients, health professionals and the public with authoritative, robust and reliable guidance on current "best practice".

■ England – Department of Health (DOH). Online. Available HTTP: <http://www.doh.gov.uk/> (accessed: 1 April 2003).
The aim of DOH is to improve the health and well-being of people in England.

- International Chemical Safety Cards. Online. Available HTTP: <http://www.cdc.gov/niosh/ipcsneng/nengsyn.html> (accessed: 1 April 2003). This international site has information on a large number of agents.
- International Toxicity Estimates for Risk (ITER). Online. Available HTTP: <http://www.tera.org/iter/> (accessed: 1 April 2003). "ITER is a compilation of human health risk values from a number of international health organizations and independent groups."
- Chemical Safety Information from intergovernmental organizations. Online. Available HTTP: <http://www.inchem.org/> (accessed: 1 April 2003). IPCS INCHEM is a means of rapid access to internationally peer reviewed information on chemicals commonly used throughout the world, which may also occur as contaminants in the environment and food. It consolidates information from a number of intergovernmental organizations whose goal it is to assist in the sound management of chemicals.
- International Pesticide Data Sheets. Online. Available HTTP: <http://www.inchem.org/pages/pds.html> (accessed: 1 April 2003). Site has a large list of pesticide data sheets.
- International Agency for Research on Cancer (IARC). Online. Available HTTP: <http://www.iarc.fr/> (accessed: 1 April 2003). IARC's mission is to coordinate and conduct research on the causes of human cancer, the mechanisms of carcinogenesis, and to develop scientific strategies for cancer control.
- World Health Organization (WHO). Online. Available HTTP: <http://www.who.int/en/> (accessed: 1 April 2003). The World Health Organization, the United Nations specialized agency for health, was established on 7 April 1948. WHO's objective, as set out in its Constitution, is the attainment by all peoples of the highest possible level of health. Information is in English, Spanish, and French.
- International Programme on Chemical Safety (IPCS). Online. Available HTTP: <http://www.who.int/pcs/index.htm> (accessed: 1 April 2003). IPCS is a joint programme of three cooperating organizations – ILO, UNEP, and WHO, implementing activities related to chemical safety.
- Encyclopaedia of Occupational Health and Safety. Online. Available HTTP: <http://www.ilocis.org/> (accessed: 1 April 2003). Published by the International Labour Organization's Constitution to promote "the protection of the worker from sickness, disease and injury arising out of employment".
- European Environment Agency. Online. Available HTTP: <http://www.eea.eu.int/> (accessed: 1 April 2003). Site has information on improving Europe's environment.
- Global Information Network on Chemicals (GINC). Online. Available HTTP: <http://www.nihs.go.jp/GINC/> (accessed: 1 April 2003). GINC is a worldwide information network for safe use of chemicals.
- EcoNet – Institute for Global Communications (IGC). Online. Available HTTP: <http://www.igc.org/> (accessed: 1 April 2003). EcoNet is part of IGC and was the world's first computer network dedicated to environmental preservation and sustainability.

- Human and Environmental Risk Assessment (HERA) – <http://www.heraproject.com/> (accessed: 1 April 2003).
  HERA is a voluntary industry program to carry out Human and Environmental Risk Assessments on ingredients of household cleaning products. HERA is a unique European partnership established in 1999 between the makers of household cleaning products (AISE) and the chemical industry (CEFIC) that supplies the raw materials.
- Australian Institute of Health and Welfare. Online. Available HTTP: <http://www.aihw.gov.au/> (accessed: 5 April 2003).
  This is Australia's national agency for health and welfare statistics and information.
- Japan – Ministry of Health, Labour and Welfare (MHLW). Online. Available HTTP: <http://www.mhlw.go.jp/english/> (accessed: 5 April 2003).
  Japan's MHLW regulates drug, food and labor safety.
- Japan – National Institute of Health Sciences (NIHS). Online. Available HTTP: <http://www.nihs.go.jp/index.html> (accessed: 5 April 2003).
  Japan's NIHS regulates drugs and chemicals.

### 1.2.3 North American agencies

- Health Canada. Online. Available HTTP: <http://www.hc-sc.gc.ca/> (accessed: 8 April 2003).
  Health Canada provides extensive health related information in English or French.
- The Canadian Centre for Occupational Health and Safety (CCOHS). Online. Available HTTP: <http://www.ccohs.ca/> (accessed: 1 April 2003).
  CCOHS promotes a safe and healthy working environment by providing information and advice about occupational health and safety.
- Canadian Health Network. Online. Available HTTP: <http://www.canadian-health-network.ca/> (accessed: 1 April 2003).
  Provides a range of health related information in both English and French. Maintained by Health Canada, of the Canadian government.
- Canadian CHEMINDEX database. Online. Available HTTP: <http://ccinfoweb.ccohs.ca/chemindex/search.html> (accessed: 1 April 2003).
  The CHEMINDEX database contains information on over 200 000 chemicals; the record contains identification information on a unique chemical substance, including chemical names and synonyms, the CAS registry number, and a list of the CCINFO databases containing information on that substance.
- Canadian MSDS Database. Online. Available HTTP: <http://ccinfoweb.ccohs.ca/msds/search.html> (accessed: 1 April 2003).
  Material Safety Data Sheets on over 120 000 compounds from 600 North American manufacturers and suppliers.
- US National Library of Medicine. Online. Available HTTP: <http://www.nlm.nih.gov/nlmhome.html> (accessed: 1 April 2003).
  This site provides access to probably the greatest sources of reference material in the world. The Health Information section has specific areas related to toxicology as well as many searchable databases.

- US Environmental Protection Agency (EPA). Online. Available HTTP: <http://www.epa.gov/> (accessed: 1 April 2003).
  Contains a wealth of information on many common environmental pollutants such as lead, mercury, and pesticides as well as regulatory information. The site also has a great children's section.
- US Environmental Protection Agency (EPA) – Integrated Risk Information System (IRIS). Online. Available HTTP: <http://www.epa.gov/iriswebp/iris/> (accessed: 1 April 2003).
  "IRIS is a database of human health effects that may result from exposure to various substances found in the environment." An excellent source of information about many compounds – a great starting place.
- US Environmental Protection Agency – Toxics Release Inventory (TRI) Program (EPA). Online. Available HTTP: <http://www.epa.gov/tri/> (accessed: 1 April 2003).
  "The Toxics Release Inventory (TRI) is a publicly available EPA database that contains information on toxic chemical releases and other waste management activities reported annually by certain covered industry groups as well as federal facilities."
- US Food and Drug Administration (FDA). Online. Available HTTP: <http://www.fda.gov/> (accessed: 1 April 2003).
  All you would ever want to know about the drug approval process as well as basic information on diseases and current event topics.
- US Food and Drug Administration (FDA) – FDA History. Online. Available HTTP: <http://www.fda.gov/opacom/backgrounders/miles.html> (accessed: 1 April 2003).
  Site contains an interesting historical perspective on the US FDA.
- US Occupational Safety and Health Administration (OSHA). Online. Available HTTP: <http://www.osha.gov> (accessed: 1 April 2003).
  OSHA is responsible for regulating the workplace environment. The site has information on current standards and business requirements.
- US National Institute for Occupational Safety and Health (NIOSH). Online. Available HTTP: <http://www.cdc.gov/niosh/> (accessed: 1 April 2003).
  NIOSH is responsible for conducting research and making recommendations for the prevention of work related disease and injury.
- US Centers for Disease Control and Prevention (CDC). Online. Available HTTP: <http://www.cdc.gov/> (accessed: 1 April 2003).
  CDC is recognized as the lead federal agency for protecting the health and safety of people of the United States.
- US Consumer Product Safety Commission (CPSC). Online. Available HTTP: <http://www.cpsc.gov/> (accessed: 1 April 2003).
  CPSC works to save lives and keep families safe by reducing the risk of injuries and deaths associated with consumer products.
- US National Toxicology Program (NTP). Online. Available HTTP: <http://ntp-server.niehs.nih.gov/> (accessed: 1 April 2003).
  NTP was established in 1978 by the Department of Health and Human Services (DHHS) to coordinate toxicological testing programs within the

Department; strengthen the science base in toxicology; develop and validate improved testing methods; and provide information about potentially toxic chemicals to health regulatory and research agencies, the scientific and medical communities, and the public.

■ US National Institute of Environmental Health Sciences (NIEHS). Online. Available HTTP: <http://www.niehs.nih.gov/> (accessed: 1 April 2003). Wide range of information linking the environment, toxicology and health.

■ California Environmental Protection Agency (CalEPA). Online. Available HTTP: <http://www.calepa.ca.gov/> (accessed: 1 April 2003). "The CalEPA mission is to restore, protect and enhance the environment, to ensure public health, environmental quality and economic vitality."

■ California Office of Environmental Health Hazard Assessment (OEHHA). Online. Available HTTP: <http://www.oehha.ca.gov/> (accessed: 1 April 2003). "The OEHHA mission is to protect and enhance public health and the environment by objective scientific evaluation of risks posed by hazardous substances."

## 1.2.4 Non-government organizations

■ Environmental Defense. Online. Available HTTP: <http://www.environmentaldefense.org/> (accessed: 1 April 2003). "Environmental Defense is dedicated to protecting the environmental rights of all people, including future generations. Among these rights are clean air and water, healthy and nourishing food, and a flourishing ecosystem."

■ Environmental Defense – Scorecard. Online. Available HTTP: <http://www.scorecard.org/> (accessed: 1 April 2003). Site has information on health effects and state exposure issues.

■ Toxicology Excellence For Risk Assessment. Online. Available HTTP: <http://www.tera.org/> (accessed: 1 April 2003). "TERA is a nonprofit (501(c)(3)) corporation dedicated to the best use of toxicity data for the development of risk values."

■ North American Association for Environmental Education (NAAEE). Online. Available HTTP: <http://www.naaee.org/> (accessed: 1 April 2003). NAAEE is a network of professionals, students, and volunteers working in the field of environmental education throughout North America and in over 55 countries around the world. Since 1971, the Association has promoted environmental education and supported the work of environmental educators.

■ American Lung Association (ALA). Online. Available HTTP: <http://www.lungusa.org/data/> (accessed: 1 April 2003). ALA fights lung disease in all its forms, with special emphasis on asthma, tobacco control, and environmental health.

■ Society of Toxicology. Online. Available HTTP: www.toxicology.org> (accessed: 1 April 2003).

■ Drug Library. Online. Available HTTP: <http://www.druglibrary.org> (accessed: 1 April 2003). Offers an incredible history and information on commonly used recreational drugs.

### 1.2.5 Library references

■ US TOXNET – National Library of Medicine. Online. Available HTTP: <http://toxnet.nlm.nih.gov/> (accessed: 1 April 2003).
TOXNET is a cluster of databases on toxicology, hazardous chemicals, and related areas.

■ US Toxicology and Environmental Health – National Library of Medicine. Online. Available HTTP: <http://sis.nlm.nih.gov/Tox/ToxMain.html> (accessed: 1 April 2003).
Site has links to many sites on a variety of toxicology information.

■ US National Library of Medicine. Online. Available HTTP: <http://www.nlm.nih.gov/> (accessed: 1 April 2003).
Site provides easy access to medical and scientific literature and numerous databases.

### 1.2.6 Introductions to toxicology and risk

■ *The Dose Makes the Poison: A Plain Language Guide to Toxicology*, by Alice Ottoboni, 1991. Van Nos Reinhold, $24.95. (A very good introduction to toxicology.)

■ *Beating Murphy's Law: The Amazing Science of Risk*, by Bob Berger, 1994. Dell, $11.95. (A fun look at risk in everyday life.)

■ *Risk Analysis and Management*, by Morgan, M. Granger. *Scientific American*, July 1993, pp. 32–41. (This is a good short overview of many of the issues in risk analysis.)

■ *Basics of Toxicology*, by Chris Kent, 1998. John Wiley & Sons, Inc., New York, 401pp. (More detailed overview but still accessible.)

### 1.2.7 Reference books (lots of good information, but costly)

■ *Principles and Methods of Toxicology*, (4th edition), ed. A. Wallace Hayes, 2001. Taylor & Francis, London, 1887 pp. (An important book on the principles of toxicology with an emphasis on testing and safety assessment in toxicology.)

■ *Casarett & Doull's Toxicology, The Basic Science of Poisons* (6th edition), ed. Curtis D. Klaassen, 2001. McGraw-Hill, New York, 1236pp. (One of the classic toxicology textbooks that contains more than anyone wants to know about toxicology.)

■ *Goodman and Gilman's The Pharmacological Basis of Therapeutics* (8th edition), ed. Joel G. Hardman, Lee E. Limbird, Perry B. Molinoff, and Raymond W. Ruddon, 1996. McGraw Hill, New York, 1905pp. (A detailed book on the pharmacological (i.e. beneficial) and toxicological (i.e. adverse) effects of drugs. Also considerable basic physiological information.)

■ US Congress, Office of Technology Assessment, *Neurotoxicity: Identifying and Controlling Poisons of the Nervous System*, OTA-BA-436 (Washington, DC: US Government Printing Office, April 1990.) (An excellent overview of toxicology with an obvious emphasis on chemical agents that affect the nervous system.)

# Chapter 2

## Principles of toxicology

### Contents

- Introduction
- Dose–response
- Demonstrating dose–response
- Hazard and risk
- Routes of exposure and absorption
- Metabolism, distribution, and excretion
- Sensitivity, susceptibility, and variability
- Applying the principles
- Summary
- Slide presentation

## 2.1 Introduction

There are three basic and interwoven principles of toxicology:

(1) dose–response
(2) hazard × exposure = risk
(3) individual sensitivity.

While these principles may form much of the foundation of toxicology, when it comes to any specific substance there is likely to be controversy. Disagreement may arise on the relative importance of any one of these principles while trying to evaluate implications for public health. Exploring these principles is an essential first step before examining their application to any specific substance. This chapter will explore some of the details and issues surrounding these principles, but first it is appropriate to put them in historical context.

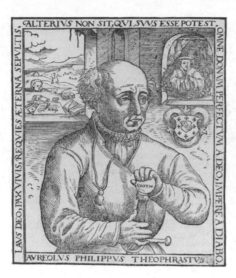

**Figure 2.1.** Paracelsus. In this portrait Paracelsus is surrounded by various philosophical symbols. From Paracelsus: *Etliche Tractaten, zum ander Mal in Truck auszgangen. Vom Podagra und seinem Speciebus* (Coln, 1567), with permission from Bernard Becker Medical Library, Washington University School of Medicine, St. Louis, USA.

Our ancient ancestors worried about being poisoned either accidentally or on purpose. The formal study of poisons (and thus toxicology) began 500 years ago during the Renaissance, a period of incredible change and challenge to traditional thought. Phillippus Aureolus (Figure 2.1), was born in Switzerland, a year after Columbus sailed in 1493. He took the pseudonym of Theophrastus Bombastus von Hohenheim and still later invented the name Paracelsus (1493–1541). This name may signify his desire to move beyond the Roman philosopher and medical writer Aulus Cornelius Celsus (c. AD 3–64), who promoted cleanliness and recommended the washing of wounds with an antiseptic such as vinegar. Paracelsus's claim to toxicology is that he elegantly stated the principle of dose–response as "All substances are poisons; there is none, which is not a poison. The right dose differentiates a poison from a remedy". This often-used quote accurately states that too much of anything, even drinking too much water, can be harmful. (It should be noted that too little of some substances can also be harmful.)

What Paracelsus failed to emphasize is the variation in sensitivity of the individual. A bee sting or a peanut can be deadly for some individuals while only annoying or even tasty for most people. There are now numerous examples demonstrating that the developing infant is very sensitive to the poisonous effects of a substance that does not harm the adult. For example, alcohol consumption during pregnancy can result in permanent harm to the infant without affecting the mother. The brain of the developing infant is sensitive to low levels of lead exposure, which is not the case for the adult. Another approach to the principle of dose–response might look like this: "The sensitivity of the individual differentiates a poison from a remedy. The fundamental principle of toxicology is the individual's response to a dose." The principle of dose–response is only useful when linked to the sensitivity of the individual.

Individual sensitivity to a hazardous agent depends on age, genetics, gender, current or prior illness, nutrition, and current or history of exposure to chemical agents. Age is an important factor for the very young or the elderly for very different reasons. The developing nervous system of the infant is more susceptible than the mature nervous system to a range of agents. Our metabolism of agents slows as we age and our bodies again become more vulnerable to the effects of an agent. Our gender and genetics dictate our ability to metabolize agents either more quickly or even not at all. For example, some people metabolize alcohol more slowly that other people because of their genetics. All these factors are important as we judge our susceptibility to a particular hazard.

There are many familiar hazards in our lives, some easier to evaluate than others. An agent or situation is hazardous when it can produce an adverse or undesirable effect. Hazard is a property of a particular agent or situation. Early in our lives we learn about the hazards of crossing the street or falling off a ladder or stumbling down the stairs. Learning about the hazards of a chemical agent is not so easy. Defining the hazard of a chemical agent requires experience in human exposures or careful study in experimental models. Through personal experience we gain an understanding of the hazards of some agents like alcohol or caffeine.

We routinely combine our knowledge of hazard, exposure, and individual susceptibility to judge the possibility or risk of harm. A young person judges the speed of the approaching car and decides to run across the street while an elderly person waits for the traffic light to change. This decision is based on a judgment about the risk of being struck by the car. An experienced mountain climber will judge the risk of harm on a difficult climb very differently from someone with no experience. Judging the risk of harm from a chemical agent is often far more difficult because the adverse effects may not be immediately obvious or may depend on individual sensitivity.

The ability of an agent to damage the nervous system or to cause cancer 10 years after exposure is clearly not obvious. The formal process of determining the potential of an agent to cause harm is called risk assessment. The risk assessment process is in itself complicated and often controversial because needed data may not be available or there is conflicting information. Risk assessment is the process of combining all the known information about the hazard of an agent and making a determination of the potential for harm to people, animals, or the environment. The next step is risk management.

Risk management combines the risk assessment with economic, political, public opinion, and other considerations to determine a course of action. These judgments seldom satisfy everyone. The principles of toxicology form the foundation for the risk assessment and ultimately for the risk management decisions. Individual and community involvement in the decision-making process is a critical part of developing sound policies to minimize risks to people and the environment.

## 2.2 Dose–response

The two most important words in toxicology are dose and response; in other words, how much of an agent will produce what reaction. In toxicology the focus is usually on adverse reaction or response, but it is equally useful to consider a full range of responses from desirable to undesirable. Experience teaches us how to moderate the dose to achieve a desired result or avoid an undesirable effect. Eating one apple is beneficial, but eating five apples may produce a stomach ache. One cup of coffee in the morning may be just right, but if you drink three cups too quickly you will suffer the consequences. For light-skinned people, acquiring a tan without getting sunburned requires careful management of exposure to the sun. While Paracelsus stated correctly that the ". . . dose differentiates a poison from a remedy", it is the individual who must constantly be aware of the dose and his or her particular response.

Defining the dose is a critical first step in the effort to predict a response. Dose is the amount of exposure to an agent, a quantitative measure of the exposure related to the subject or individual. For a chemical agent or drug the dose is the amount of the material in relation to body weight. Typically the amount of material is measured in grams or thousandths of a gram (milligrams, mg) and body weight is measured in kilograms (kg), equal to 1000 grams (g). The dose is calculated as follows:

Oral dose = amount of material consumed (mg)/body weight (kg)

By knowing just a couple of facts we can turn our everyday exposure of caffeine into a dose. There are approximately 100 mg of caffeine in a cup of coffee. The actual amount of caffeine in a cup of coffee depends on the coffee bean, how the coffee was prepared, and the size of the cup. An adult weighing 155 lbs (about 70 kg) consuming this one cup of coffee would receive a dose of 100 mg divided by 70 kg, or 1.4 mg/kg of caffeine. The importance of including body weight becomes clear if you consider a child who weighs only 5 kg (11 lbs). If this child consumed the same cup of coffee, the dose would be 100 mg/5 kg or 20 mg/kg, more than ten times higher than the adult.

The difficult part of calculating the dose is often determining the exact amount of exposure to the agent. The amount of caffeine in a cup of coffee varies depending on the bean and brewing method, to say nothing of the size of the cup. Very sensitive instrumentation is now available to analytical chemists to determine accurately the amount of a specific agent in a material. If the agent is pure, it is relatively easy to determine the amount of the substance and then calculate the dose. Some foods, such as table salt or sugar, are relatively pure and the dose easily calculated by weighing the material. Package labeling usually indicates how many milligrams of the drug each pill contains, so the dose can be calculated. An infant formulation contains much less drug per pill, but because of the difference in weight between the infant and the adult the dose is similar.

Calculating the dose following workplace or environmental exposure can be far more difficult. If the agent is in the air, then calculation of the dose must consider not only the concentration in the air but also the duration of the exposure, rate of breathing, and body weight. The amount of air inhaled over a period of time is estimated from laboratory data. Given this information, it is possible to estimate the dose according to the following formula:

$$\text{Inhalation dose (mg/kg)} = \text{air concentration of agent (mg/ml)}$$
$$\times \text{volume of air inhaled per hour (ml/h)}$$
$$\times \text{duration of exposure (h)/body weight (kg)}$$

For non-chemical exposures, other variables and different units of measurement are required. For example, exposure to sunlight could be measured in hours, but to determine the dose would require knowing the intensity of the light as well as the exposed skin surface area.

Workplace and environmental exposures are often repeated and ongoing over an extended period of time. The health effects of repeated long-term exposures can be very different from one short-term exposure.

Duration of exposure, frequency of exposure and time between exposures are important determinants of dose and response. Four beers in one hour would produce a very different response than four beers over four days. Many years of repeated high levels of alcohol exposure can lead to serious liver damage as well as other health complications quite different from the short-term consequences of one exposure to a high level of alcohol. Acute exposure is a single or very limited number of exposures over a short period of time. Chronic exposure is repeated exposure over a long period of time. The effects of acute or chronic exposure, as in the case of alcohol, are often very different. For many drugs we are looking for the immediate or acute response following exposure. We consume common painkillers with the desire to stop our headache quickly. Long-term repeated use, however, can have undesirable effects on the stomach or liver. Tobacco users desire the acute effect of the nicotine but can suffer the chronic effects of long-term use such as lung cancer and heart disease. It is also possible to have a delayed response to an acute exposure. For example, a laboratory researcher died several months after an acute exposure to a small amount of ethyl mercury. Detailed knowledge about the hazards of a substance is necessary in evaluating exposure and effect or dose–response relationships. This includes information about the consequences of acute or chronic exposure.

There is often a range of responses associated with any particular agent. The response that occurs will vary with the dose, the duration of exposure, and the individual. The acute response to a single dose is often the easiest to characterize, but the response to multiple exposures over a long period of time may be the most important. An emergency response worker who is exposed acutely to a solvent in the air may have her or his judgment impaired, resulting in a serious mistake. However, over the long term this exposure is of no consequence, assuming the worker survives any mistake in judgment. On the other hand, long-term exposure to coal dust can lead to black lung and severe disability. For a long time it was thought that the only serious complication from childhood lead exposure was death resulting from high exposure. Subsequent research demonstrated that even small amounts of lead exposure during childhood could result in brain damage that lasts a lifetime. Determining what responses are most important is a central aspect of many debates in toxicology.

## 2.3 Demonstrating dose–response

In general, it is true that for any individual, the greater the dose the greater the response. This concept is illustrated in Figure 2.2 and can be easily demonstrated in the home or classroom with a few simple items (see Appendix – Dose–response demonstration). Caffeine, which distributes evenly throughout total body water, is a good illustration of dose–response. It is important to know if a substance distributes into body water because we are made up of approximately 75% water. A can of cola contains approximately 50 mg of caffeine (about 4 mg per ounce of cola). Consumption of the first can of cola delivers an exposure of 50 mg per total body weight. Assuming a 100 kg person, this would be 50/100 mg/kg or 0.5 mg/kg. Consumption of three cans of cola would result in a dose of 1.5 mg/kg and six cans of cola a dose of 3 mg/kg of caffeine. Because caffeine distributes evenly throughout body water you can almost imagine the change in shade depicted in Figure 2.2 as the concentration of the caffeine in the blood. An individual's response to the caffeine varies with the dose and corresponding amount of circulating caffeine.

The right panel (Figure 2.2) illustrates the effect of body size on the dose. When the adult and the child receive the same amount of caffeine, the exposure is the same but the dose is dramatically different. A child who weighs only 10 kg

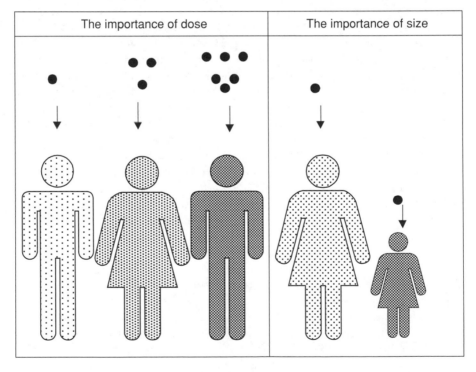

**Figure 2.2.** The effect of dose and body size on response. For a given body size, the larger dose produces a greater effect (left), and for a given exposure, the smaller body size receives a greater effect and larger dose (right).

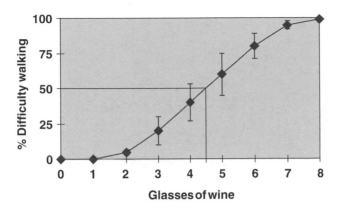

**Figure 2.3.** Dose–response graph for drinking wine. Dose–response function for difficulty in walking and number of glasses of wine consumed. This is an idealized curve, but it illustrates the principle that at low doses (i.e. few glasses) there is little response, then an increasing response to a maximum response. Note that this figure does not take into consideration body weight or any other variables such as gender or frequency of exposure (i.e. time between drinks).

receives a dose of 5 mg/kg after one can of cola. An adult who weighs 100 kg must drink 10 cans of cola to receive an equivalent dose. Body size is a critical factor in determining dose and any subsequent response. For the equivalent exposure to any substance such as lead or a pesticide, the child will receive a much greater dose than the adult. As we shall discover, there are other important physiological factors that also make children more susceptible than adults to the effects of an agent.

The next figure (Figure 2.3) graphically illustrates the critical relationship between dose and response. In this case, we define the response as difficulty in walking and the dose of or exposure to alcohol as a glass of wine. To change from exposure to dose we would need to know the body weight and amount of alcohol in the glass of wine. If we selected a group of people at random and offered them wine, no one (most likely) would have difficulty walking after one drink (depending of course on how big the glass was). The number of people responding, or in this case having difficulty walking, is a percentage of the total number of people in our study population. As exposure to wine increases, more and more people would have difficultly walking until finally everyone was affected. In toxicology, the dose at which one half or 50% of the population is affected is often calculated and used to compare the toxicity of different agents. In this example, 50% of the population is affected after exposure to 4.5 glasses of wine. The vertical bars represent the variability from one test group to the next. If we repeat this experiment with a different group of people, the actual data points could be somewhat different, but should generally fall within the range spanned by the vertical bars or error bars. There are many possible reasons for this variation, including body weight (which changes dose), food consumption prior to drinking, past use of alcohol, genetics, gender, as well as others. Technically this figure is an exposure–response graph because

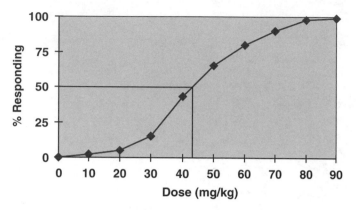

**Figure 2.4.** An idealized dose–response graph. The horizontal axis indicates the dose in mg/kg of body weight, while the vertical axis is the percent of maximum response. For a very low dose there is no or little response. The response increases with the dose until the maximum response is reached and increasing the dose has no additional effect.

the dose is not calculated; the number of glasses of wine represents a measure of exposure not dose.

Figure 2.4 demonstrates an "S"-shaped idealized dose–response graph, which is typical of most types of exposure. In this figure the percentage responding is plotted against the dose in mg/kg. This "S"-shaped curve illustrates that at low doses there is little or no response while at high doses all individuals respond or demonstrate the effect. The line drawn at 50% responses determines at what dose 50% of the population would demonstrate this response. In this situation, 50% of the subjects respond at a dose of 42 mg/kg, while 99% of the subjects responded at 90 mg/kg. It is important to emphasize that if we repeat this experiment the results would be slightly different. Each individual varies from one time to the next and there is even greater variability between individuals. Variability is a consistent theme in biology, complicating data analysis and interpretation of results. These variations lead to the need for statistical evaluation of data.

## 2.4 Hazard and risk

The biological effects of an agent often span a broad range from beneficial to harmful, depending on the dose and individual sensitivity. The scientific discipline of toxicology was developed in an effort to understand and characterize the potentially harmful or hazardous properties of an agent. Risk is the probability of injury, disease, loss of function, or death for an individual or population exposed to a hazardous substance or situation. An agent or situation that can produce or cause a harmful or adverse effect is a hazard. Hazard is an intrinsic property of a substance and any particular substance may have a range of hazards associated with it depending upon specific conditions or circumstances. On a daily basis, we routinely confront a range of potentially hazardous agents, including the fire we cook with, the electricity that lights our homes, the household chemicals used for cleaning, the chemicals that run our cars, drugs in the medicine we take, and the list goes on. We use these potentially hazardous agents but are careful to avoid conditions that will result in the expression of their hazardous properties. Gasoline is a good example of an agent with multiple hazards. We depend on its flammability to make our cars run but that same flammability can be hazardous in an uncontrolled fire. Sniffing gasoline, undertaken by some people for effects on the nervous system, represents a very different hazard. Problems develop when we do not fully appreciate an agent's potential to cause harm or the conditions under which the agent can cause harm. Problems can also occur when products or mechanical systems malfunction.

In the past, the hazard associated with any particular substance was related to immediate or obvious harm. As our knowledge and experience increase, so too does our appreciation of an agent's ability to produce unexpected consequences or harm. Take for example DDT, a very powerful pesticide useful in the eradication of mosquitoes. As Rachel Carson so eloquently pointed out, DDT devastated bird populations not directly but indirectly by thinning eggshells to such an extent that the eggshells failed. This resulted in a devastating decline in bird populations, particularly for birds consuming animals. Still later we learned that DDT was a very persistent chemical and highly soluble in fat. DDT thus accumulated up the food chain and in this case birds at the top of the food chain were most affected. Humans are also at the top of the food chain, and through a variety of means, DDT ends up in the food supply and becomes stored in body fat. When women are breast-feeding, fat and DDT are mobilized and become the food of nursing infants, which represents a large dose to a small infant. We are still unsure of the consequences of fetal exposure to DDT and its effects on the developing organism. Many other fat-soluble chemicals, such as dioxin and polychlorinated biphenyls (PCBs) are known to contaminate breast milk. Lead is another example of a major public health disaster that occurred because the consequences of low-level lead exposure to the developing nervous system were not appreciated.

Recognition of the potential harmful effects of agents from drugs to pesticides resulted in new research efforts as well as the formation of government agencies responsible for regulating hazardous substances. The US Food and Drug Administration (FDA) is responsible for ensuring that all drugs and food additives are both efficacious and safe. The Occupational Health and Safety Administration (OSHA) establishes rules to control or limit exposures to a variety of chemicals in the workplace, based upon toxicology data. The Consumer Products Safety Commission (CPSC) works to reduce injury from consumer products. The US Environmental Protection Agency (EPA) governs the release of chemicals into the environment to protect the soil, water, and air. It also regulates the clean-up of hazardous chemicals in the environment.

While science plays an important role in characterizing the harmful effects of an agent, society also establishes laws to regulate or limit exposure to known hazards. Tobacco and alcohol consumption are legal despite recognized hazards and considerable cost to society. It was only recently that the government forced the tobacco industry into acknowledging the addictive properties of nicotine and began to recover health costs through litigation. While the adverse effects of excessive alcohol consumption have been recognized for a long time, it was only in the 1970s that birth defects related to alcohol consumption during pregnancy were recognized. In contrast, the US government has declared that marijuana and many other recreational drugs are illegal based upon their known hazard characteristics. Obviously, this is a controversial area, with many people (and even countries) having very different opinions and laws.

Hazard and risk are linked by exposure. Reducing the hazard, the exposure, or both can lower risk. If there is no exposure, then there is no risk or possibility of harm. Knowledge and experience allow one to judge the potential for harm or risk associated with exposure to a substance. In this way we are all toxicologists, always judging the potential for harm against the benefit of exposure. This is often easier said than done, but being knowledgeable about an agent can lead to the development of specific strategies to reduce the potential for harm. Since one cannot necessarily foresee all possible exposures to a hazardous substance, choosing less hazardous substances is also a vital part of risk reduction.

The beneficial use of radiation is one of the best examples of how careful characterization of the hazard is essential for its safe use. A radioactive substance can be safely stored or transported if appropriately contained. Depending on the characteristics of the radioactive material, it can be safely handled by using appropriate shielding and safety precautions. Laboratory workers usually wear special badges that quantify radiation exposure to ensure that predetermined levels of exposure, which are considered safe, are not exceeded. Unfortunately, after more than 50 years, society has not yet been able to design and implement a safe way to dispose of radioactive waste. The hazardous properties of radiation are explored further in a subsequent chapter.

Historically, potentially toxic agents have been ranked by their lethality, or the amount of material that causes death. In this measure, hazard is defined only as death, obviously only the grossest measure of an agent's effect. Because of individual variability or susceptibility, a standardized measure is the dose (in units of mg/kg) that produces death in half of the subjects, a 50% response. This is called an $LD_{50}$ or lethal dose for 50% of the population. The $LD_{50}$ is one measure of the *toxicity* of a substance, its capacity for causing illness or death. The $LD_{50}$ is usually determined on populations of test animals such as rats and mice. Determination of an $LD_{50}$ is based on a single acute exposure to an agent and the single response of death. Although the $LD_{50}$ can be useful in comparing the gross hazards of agents, it is not necessarily relevant to a response produced by low-level chronic exposure. For example, the $LD_{50}$ of lead is not particularly important, given its adverse effects on the developing nervous system even at very low levels of exposure. $LD_{50}$s are misleading if used as the only characterization of the toxicity of a substance. Aspirin is a commonly used over-the-counter medicine, while DDT is a pesticide that has been banned because of its toxic effects and persistence in the environment, yet they have similar $LD_{50}$s.

Table 2.1 lists the $LD_{50}$s of a variety of common agents. Since the $LD_{50}$ is the amount of material required to produce death, a higher $LD_{50}$ implies a lower toxicity and vice versa. Note how high the $LD_{50}$ is for alcohol, which is fortunate given its widespread consumption. This explains why so few people die as a result of acute alcohol consumption. Generally, people pass out at high blood alcohol levels and do not die directly as a result of the alcohol but from suffocating on

**Table 2.1 Approximate acute LD$_{50}$s of some common chemical agents**

| Agent | LD$_{50}$ (mg/kg) |
| --- | --- |
| Ethyl alcohol | 10,000 |
| Salt (sodium chloride) | 4,000 |
| Iron (ferrous sulfate) | 1,500 |
| Morphine | 900 |
| Mothballs (paradichlorobenzene) | 500 |
| Aspirin | 250 |
| DDT | 250 |
| Cyanide | 10 |
| Nicotine | 1 |
| Tetrodotoxin (from fish) | 0.01 |
| Dioxin (TCDD) | 0.001 (for some species) |
| Botulinum toxin | 0.00001 |

their own vomit as the body tries to rid itself of this toxicant. Note also the low LD$_{50}$ (high toxicity) for nicotine, the most active and addictive ingredient in cigarettes.

Fortunately, the LD$_{50}$ is no longer recognized as an adequate or even particularly useful assessment of an agent's ability to cause harm. Toxicologists have developed a wide array of tests to determine if an agent can produce an adverse effect. A variety of tests are performed to evaluate the potential harmful effects across all organ systems. If any hint of adverse effects is observed, further testing is done to characterize and understand the effect thoroughly. Ultimately, the hazard must be judged on the sensitivity of the individual. Moderate consumption of alcohol can present few hazards for an adult, but this same amount of alcohol can harm the developing fetus. Lead has many beneficial uses and has long been recognized as a hazard, but it is only relatively recently that harmful effects on the developing nervous system have been characterized. At what point does caffeine produce an undesirable effect and another cup of coffee become something to avoid? How much of a hazard is caffeine? To answer these questions, we need to know more about how the body metabolizes or breaks down chemical agents.

## 2.5 Routes of exposure and absorption

An agent exerts its effects when it enters or comes into contact with the body, in other words, when an individual has been exposed to it. Although we are primarily concerned with effects on humans, the same principles apply to all living organisms and, indeed, to the entire environment. *Exposure*, like many of the terms in toxicology, has several difference aspects, the most important of which are:

(1) route of exposure
(2) frequency of exposure
(3) duration of exposure.

Exposure is also affected by absorption. Even though we may come into contact with an agent, if little is taken up into the body (or absorbed), there is little effect. For example, the metallic mercury from a broken thermometer, if swallowed, is very poorly absorbed by the gut and will be excreted in the feces. However, if this same amount of mercury were allowed to evaporate and be inhaled, there would be very serious health consequences. This example shows that metabolism and excretion modify absorption. What is not absorbed (and even some of what is absorbed) may be excreted from the body by various routes, including the urine, feces, and sweat or through exhalation. Excretion reduces the effect because it lowers the amount of toxicant in the body, thus reducing exposure to sensitive organs.

There are three main routes of exposure:

(1)  skin (or dermal) exposure
(2)  lung (inhalation) exposure
(3)  oral (gastrointestinal) exposure.

A fourth route of exposure is by injection, which is used for delivery of drugs or medication that cannot be taken orally. Injections can take several forms. An injection directly into a blood vessel (intravenously or IV) bypasses most of the absorption barriers and the drug will have almost full and immediate access to most organs of the body. Some medications are injected into the muscle (intramuscularly or IM), which slows absorption as the drug is gradually taken up by the blood supplying the muscle. Finally, injections can be made just under the skin (subcutaneous or SC). This method is commonly used for allergy testing or tuberculin (TB) tests.

Skin is the largest organ of the body and does an amazing job of protecting us from most agents. However, the skin is an important route of exposure to some agents and also a site of highly adverse reactions. For example, the adverse effect of too much exposure to the sun is well known. In many cases, the skin is an excellent barrier to chemical agents, but some solvents can readily penetrate the skin. Solvents such as gasoline or chemical cleaners can easily remove the natural oils of the skin and result in adverse skin reaction, as well as chemical absorption. The labels of many pesticides state that gloves and other skin protection should be worn because of the risk of pesticide absorption through the skin or allergic reaction such as a rash. A number of medications can now be applied through a skin patch, such as nicotine patches to curb the desire to smoke cigarettes. The advantage of a skin patch is that the drug will be absorbed at a constant slow rate, thus keeping the drug blood levels relatively constant. This system helps smokers by keeping their blood nicotine levels elevated and constant, curbing the desire to smoke.

Inhalation is an excellent route of exposure to many agents, including the oxygen essential for life. The lungs are very rich in blood to facilitate the absorption of oxygen and thus allow the rapid absorption of other agents directly into the bloodstream, quickly producing an effect. Carbon monoxide is a potentially lethal gas that can be generated in the home by poorly ventilated heaters, faulty furnaces, or a car idling in an attached garage. Carbon monoxide is readily taken up by the blood cells by the same mechanism as oxygen. In fact, carbon monoxide binds to the hemoglobin in the blood cells better than oxygen, so exposure can cause serious injury and even death through lack of oxygen intake. Cigarette smokers become dependent on the nicotine absorbed through the lungs from the tobacco smoke. Marijuana users hold their breath to allow additional absorption of the active ingredient THC. The lungs can also excrete some agents, although this is usually in very small amounts. The excretion of alcohol forms the basis for the alcohol Breathalyzer test, which quantifies the amount of alcohol in the body by measuring what is exhaled.

Ingestion of substances orally allows absorption from the stomach and intestines. This is a critical route of exposure for many agents, from essential carbohydrates, proteins, and vitamins, to unwanted pesticides and lead. All that is ingested is not necessarily absorbed, and absorption can be dependent on age. For example, in an adult, only about 10% of the lead ingested is absorbed, but up to 50% may be absorbed by an infant or pregnant woman. In this case, unabsorbed lead is passed through the intestine and excreted in the feces. The increased absorption of certain agents at different times of life is related to the body's demand for important elements. In this situation, the intestines are able to absorb increased amounts of calcium and iron but will take lead as a poor substitute (more on this in the lead chapter). Alcohol and caffeine are readily absorbed by the stomach, making for two of the most popular drugs in our culture. Oral exposure also occurs through our food and drinking water, so it is imperative to have unpolluted water and a safe food supply. It is also a good idea to wash your hands before eating or touching food so that what may be on your skin is not transferred to the food you eat.

The other two aspects of exposure are frequency and duration. Frequency can refer not only to the number of times the exposure occurred, but also to the time between exposures. For example, drinking four beers within 15 minutes is quite different from drinking four beers in four days. Frequent exposure of a short duration results in rapidly elevated blood levels of any agent (assuming it's absorbed). Two quick cups of coffee in the morning serve to elevate blood caffeine levels, whereas slowly sipping a cup of coffee will not have the desired stimulator effect. It takes approximately 30 minutes to absorb the caffeine from a cup of coffee and reach your peak blood caffeine levels. The harmful or toxic effects of an agent are often dependent on the frequency of exposure and the time between exposures.

Duration of exposure is a closely related factor. In toxicology, duration is usually divided into three periods:

(1) acute exposure (usually just one or two exposures of short duration)
(2) subchronic exposure (multiple exposures over many days or perhaps months)
(3) chronic exposure (long-term or even lifetime exposure).

The terms acute and chronic are also used to characterize the time delay between exposure and the onset of symptoms. Acute effects are those noticed directly following exposure and are usually easily related to the agent. The chronic or long-term effects of an agent may occur years later and are often very difficult to attribute to a particular cause. The acute effects of alcohol consumption or exposure to the solvent in glue are obvious in the drunkenness produced. The effects of chronic exposure to these compounds, as seen by an alcoholic, are very different: specifically, cirrhosis of the liver. The chronic effect of childhood lead exposure can be impaired learning that will be a factor throughout an individual's lifetime. The chronic effects of food additives and pesticides are evaluated in lifetime animal studies to assess the carcinogenic (cancer-causing) potential of these agents.

There are two types of exposure that deserve special attention: fetal exposure during pregnancy and exposure of the brain. For a long time it was thought that the placenta offered the developing fetus significant protection from hazardous agents. We know now that the majority of agents readily cross the placenta and expose the developing fetus to whatever the mother has been exposed to. The fluid surrounding the infant (amniotic fluid) will have the same level of drug as the mother's blood for compounds that readily distribute throughout body water, such as caffeine. Thus the infant is literally swimming in caffeine and its metabolites. Fetal methyl mercury can actually be higher than that of the mother, because the developing infant acts as a storage site for maternal mercury. The brain, on the other hand, in the adult but not in the fetus, is afforded some extra protection from hazardous agents. This barrier is known as the blood–brain barrier because of its ability to keep some agents from moving from the blood vessels into the brain tissue. This barrier works primarily on large molecules but does not stop water-soluble agents such as caffeine from entering the brain and producing its stimulatory effect. While there are obviously many good aspects of the blood–brain barrier, it has also proven to be very challenging to move desirable drugs into the brain to treat disease.

From a scientific perspective, we work primarily with single exposures to chemicals to understand how the body reacts to a specific chemical. In real life, however, we are often exposed to a mixture of chemical agents. Multiple agents may interact and affect absorption or how the body reacts to the chemical. The body has a very sophisticated system to metabolize and eliminate chemicals from the body; this system plays an important role in protecting us from hazardous substances.

## 2.6 Metabolism, distribution, and excretion

Fortunately, living organisms have developed elaborate systems to defend themselves against toxic agents. Metabolism refers to an organism's ability to change a substance into different chemical parts or metabolites that are usually less toxic. The body metabolizes the food we consume to recover energy and basic elements necessary for our well being. In toxicology, metabolism refers to the body's ability to reduce an agent into parts that are either less harmful or more readily excreted, a process called detoxification. The most common route of excretion is through urine, although some agents can be excreted in the feces, sweat, or even the breath. For toxic agents, metabolism is beneficial, but it can also reduce the benefits of a drug needed to aid in the recovery from an illness. Distribution refers to the process where an agent goes into the body. Some agents such as pesticides and PCBs accumulate in the fat. Other agents such as lead can accumulate in the bone in the place of calcium. Agents stored in the body may never be fully excreted; as we age we continue to accumulate a body burden of these stored agents like PCB or lead. Metabolism, distribution, and excretion are linked aspects that are essential in predicting the adverse effects of an agent and thus determining the risk of exposure to it.

Although most cells in the body are capable of metabolism, the primary organ for detoxification is the liver. The liver has a variety of specialized cells that produce enzymes to aid in the metabolism of toxic agents. These enzymes can break down toxic agents into smaller elements, making them less toxic. In some cases the compounds are changed so that they are more easily filtered by the kidney and excreted in the urine. Alcohol and caffeine, for example, are metabolized in the liver. The liver is a remarkable organ but can be permanently damaged by diseases such as hepatitis or through long-term alcohol consumption. Liver damage can be detected in the blood by looking for elevated levels of compounds produced by the liver. Insurance companies use liver function tests to evaluate the possibility of chronic drug consumption.

Not all agents can be readily metabolized. The toxic metals lead and mercury are elements that cannot be degraded but must still be removed from the body. Another important mechanism of detoxification is the attachment or binding of another compound to a toxic chemical to make it easier for the kidney to filter the compound out of the blood and excrete it in the urine. A primary purpose of the kidney is to screen the blood for waste products and concentrate them in the urine for excretion, as occurs, for example, with mercury. Caffeine is excreted in the urine at approximately the same concentration as the blood because the kidney cannot concentrate caffeine. Vitamins, however, are readily concentrated and excess quickly eliminated in the urine.

Chelators bind metals so that they are more readily excreted in the urine. In the past, chelators were routinely prescribed to people with elevated blood lead levels in an effort to accelerate the excretion of lead in the urine. Unless the blood levels are excessively elevated the current treatment is to determine the source of the lead exposure and take remedial action. The problem with chelators is that they are non-specific and bind useful agents such as calcium.

Half-life is a measure of the length of time an agent stays in the body before being metabolized and eliminated. More precisely, the half-life of an agent refers to the time it takes to reduce the level of the agent by one-half. For example, if the amount of caffeine in your blood was measured as 12 units (the particular units are not important), it would take approximately 5 hours for that level to be reduced to 6 units. In this case, 5 hours represents the half-life of caffeine. Another 5 hours later the amount would be reduced by half to 3 units, and so on until it approaches zero. The half-life of an agent, either toxic or beneficial, is a critical aspect of its ability to produce and maintain an effect. There can be considerable individual variability in the ability to metabolize an agent. This variability is reflected in the half-life for that particular individual. Someone who rapidly metabolizes caffeine (meaning someone for whom caffeine has a short half-life, say 3 hours) may want to drink more coffee more rapidly to elevate and maintain high caffeine blood levels and achieve the desired effect. Others may find that one cup of coffee every 3 or 4 hours is adequate. A variety of factors, such as liver disease or even pregnancy, can decrease the metabolism or excretion of an agent and thus increase the half-life. During pregnancy the half-life of caffeine increases to approximately 7 hours, resulting in higher blood caffeine levels for a longer period of time. While the half-life of agents such as caffeine and alcohol are relatively short, many of the most serious environmental toxicants have much longer half-life values. For example,

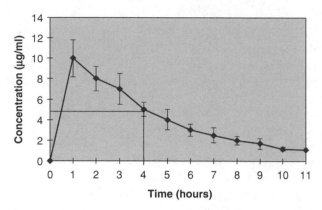

**Figure 2.5.** A characterization of half-life. A substance is consumed at time zero (for example, drink a cup of coffee and we could measure blood caffeine concentrations) and blood samples are collected hourly. Concentration of the agent is plotted against time. The black line represents the half-life when the blood concentration has dropped by one-half of its maximum. Thus, in this example, the half-life is 4 hours.

the half-life of lead is approximately 30 days. Many pesticides and PCBs are also readily stored in the body and have corresponding long half-life values. Careful consideration of the half-life of a drug is an important aspect during medical treatment. The half-life of a hypothetical drug is illustrated in Figure 2.5.

The ability of an agent to enter a specific organ of the body often dictates its effect. For example, alcohol and caffeine would not be consumed were they not readily distributed to the brain, where they produce a considerable effect. As already mentioned, lead can be exchanged for calcium and accumulate in the bone, while many pesticides and PCBs are stored in fat cells. These patterns of distribution and the storage of compounds in the body can have serious toxicological implications. During rapid weight loss, excess toxicants can be redistributed into the blood supply as fat is metabolized. Lead in the bone can also be mobilized if there is heavy demand for calcium, as occurs during pregnancy. To complicate matters further, each area of the body – in this case the fat and bone – can have its own half-life that can differ from that of blood. The half-life of lead in the blood is measured in days, while that in bone is measured in years.

## 2.7 Sensitivity, susceptibility, and variability

Susceptibility refers to the differences in sensitivity to toxic agents, causing some people to suffer greater effects than others from the same exposure. This is a key concept in toxicology and risk analysis/management. Susceptibility is primarily related to several factors, including age, sex, health, and genetic background. Sensitivity is related to susceptibility but generally refers to special cases of extreme susceptibility to certain agents by some people. Someone who is allergic to bee stings can have a fatal reaction when stung by just one bee, while for most others a sting is of little concern. Enhanced sensitivity to a compound can develop after repeated exposure to it or a similar agent. Allergies to animals such as cats and dogs are examples of specific sensitivities to an agent called animal dander. Other individuals may develop a sensitivity to dust mites.

In general the young and elderly are most susceptible to the adverse effects of an agent. The young, particularly the very young, are more susceptible because the organs are still rapidly developing, and dividing cells are more easily harmed than mature cells. For example, lead affects the developing nervous system to a much greater degree than the adult brain. The brain is rapidly growing during and after birth, particularly throughout the first 7 years of life. The brain is not fully developed until the late teens. During the first year of life the metabolism of agents by the liver is also reduced. This is why the half-life of caffeine can be measured in days for the newborn while it is hours for the adult. The elderly are more sensitive to agents because of decreased ability to metabolize them and decreased ability to compensate for the effects.

Gender can also play an important role in susceptibility to agents, in part due to hormonal influences. The classic example is the female birth control pill. In this case, a very small exposure to specific hormones has a very large influence on fertility. Other agents such as PCBs also appear to affect some of the female hormones. Some athletes use hormones called steroids to increase muscle mass. These agents have different toxic side effects for males and females. Females have additional issues related to pregnancy. Pregnancy causes many changes in physiology that can alter the absorption, distribution, and metabolism of an agent and thus dramatically influence its effects. For example, during pregnancy there is a decrease in liver metabolism that increases the half-life of caffeine. This means that a pregnant woman will maintain higher blood caffeine levels for a longer period of time than when not pregnant, resulting in increased caffeine exposure to the developing infant. Agents stored in the fat, such as pesticides and PCBs, can be mobilized during lactation and thus passed on to a nursing infant. Calcium mobilization during pregnancy can also redistribute lead from the bone if there has been previous lead exposure.

Personal health is another factor that can influence susceptibility to an agent. A compromised liver or immune system can make exposure to even low levels of an agent completely intolerable. Someone who is diabetic may find sugar toxic and may enjoy considerable benefit from artificial sweeteners. On the other hand, someone who cannot metabolize phenylalanine, a naturally occurring and essential substance, may find the common artificial sweetener in some soft drinks toxic. An individual who suffers from asthma may find exposure to wood smoke extremely harmful, whereas many people can tolerate short exposures to it fairly well. (Wood smoke is nevertheless toxic in either case, and chronic exposure can lead to health problems.) The physiological changes of disease or chronic illness are thus very important considerations in assessing the exposure to an agent.

Finally, our genetic variability may make us more or less prone to disease or the effects of a toxic agent. Some can tolerate caffeine before bed, while for others such exposure would result in a restless night. It is always important to consider the individual and the individual characteristics of a situation.

## 2.8 Applying the principles

### 2.8.1 Multiple chemical exposure

In the real world we are not exposed to only one chemical at a time. The air we breathe contains many separate chemicals. Indoor air in homes can contain chemicals from smoke, molds, carpet glue, mothballs, and cleaning products, to name only a few. Determining the risk from such multiple exposures is difficult because the body does not necessarily respond to each chemical in the mixture in the same way it would if the others were not present. Sometimes one chemical can cause the body to respond more strongly to another chemical generating a synergistic effect. We know, for example, that exposure to environmental tobacco smoke greatly increases the risk of cancer from asbestos. The increase is not additive – that is, it is not equal to the risk from tobacco plus the risk from asbestos – but is actually much greater than the sum of the two risks.

There are also cases where exposure to two chemicals reduces toxic effects. Methanol (wood alcohol) causes blindness if ingested. Methanol poisoning is treated by administering ethanol (common alcohol), which competes for metabolism in the body, thus slowing the formation of toxic byproducts of methanol and keeping their levels low enough to avoid damage to the visual system. This is sometimes referred to as an antagonistic effect.

When more than two chemicals are involved, the problem of determining risks becomes increasingly complex. Scientific study of chemical mixtures has been relatively limited because of the sheer number of combinations possible. Even if the exact effects of exposure to mixtures are unknown, reducing exposure is still a good strategy to lower risk.

### 2.8.2 Multiple chemical sensitivity

Multiple chemical sensitivity (MCS) is characterized by a variety of adverse effects upon multiple organs that result from exposure to levels of common foods, drugs, and chemicals that do not affect most people. Symptoms include headaches, fatigue, lack of concentration, memory loss, asthma, and other often subjective responses following exposure. MCS has remained controversial because standard medical evaluations, such as blood biochemical screens, have failed to identify consistent physical or laboratory test abnormalities that would account for the symptoms.

MCS is thought to develop following sensitization to one chemical, a sensitivity that then is generalized so that chemicals of a similar class and lower concentrations of exposure come to elicit the response. Researchers have been working to develop a mechanism of action for these responses and have focused on the immune system responses and, more recently, on involvement of the nervous system. Others investigators, while respecting the symptomatology, postulate that the responses are due to some form of psychological illnesses. Whatever the mechanism of action, it is important to attempt to associate cause and effect relationships and apply the principles of toxicology. Identification of what agents may be causing the symptoms can result in plans to reduce exposure to these agents and thus reduce symptoms and improve the quality of life. In addition, reductions in the exposure to toxic chemicals for all persons may help reduce the incidence of MCS.

### 2.8.3 Assessing and managing risk

As we have seen, risk is closely related to hazard and is defined as the probability of the recognized hazard occurring. Risk assessment is the process by which the nature and magnitude of risk are identified, while risk management is the process of determining whether or how much to reduce risk through our actions. Evaluation of the potential adverse effects of some activity or exposure (risk assessment) is something we all do informally on a day-to-day basis. What we decide to do is in part the result of an ongoing risk management decision. It can be as simple as crossing the street against a red light or as complex as spending the extra money for organically grown foods to reduce our exposure to pesticides. Many of the risks associated with chemical exposure are indirect or subtle effects on health; in other words, conditions, situations, or exposures to an agent that affect the quality of life. Table 2.2 lists some of the factors that can influence a person's perceptions and views about health concerns.

Risk analysis and risk management play an important role in public policy. These debates range from the development of environmental impact statements for the location of buildings to debates on household lead abatement and what chemicals can be allowed in the food supply. Quality of life issues such as asthma and/or loss of mental function are now recognized as important components of risk assessment. For example, childhood exposure to lead can result in reduced IQ, which can affect an individual throughout their lifetime. Similarly, childhood asthma can have a severe impact on an individual's ability to play and socialize.

In the past, much of the formal risk assessment concerned an estimation of the risk of cancer and subsequent death and then deciding what was acceptable.

**Table 2.2 Considerations that influence acceptability of risk**

| More-acceptable risk | Less-acceptable risk |
| --- | --- |
| Benefits understood | Benefits unclear |
| No alternatives | Alternatives available |
| Risk shared | Risk affects few |
| Voluntary | Involuntary |
| Individual control | Uncontrollable |
| Familiar | Unfamiliar |
| Low dread | High dread |
| Affects everybody | Affects children |
| Naturally occurring | Human origin (synthetic) |
| Little media attention | High media attention |
| Understood | Not understood |
| High trust | Low trust |

Typically, a risk of death of less than 1 in 100,000 ($10^{-5}$) or 1 in 1 million ($10^{-6}$) is considered an "acceptable" level of risk for exposure to a chemical. In comparison, the risk of death in an automobile accident is 1 in 4000 and the risk of death from lightning is 1 in 2 million. Comparisons like those above are sometimes used to argue that the risk of exposure to a chemical agent is negligible. Such comparisons can be misleading, however, if the conditions of the two risks are different. For example, if they affect different populations unequally, say falling disproportionately on those of a particular ethnic background, the risks may be more likely to be judged unacceptable. Or if one risk is the result of voluntary choice (drinking alcohol) and another is not (eating food contaminated with bacteria), it cannot be assumed that an individual will be equally willing to tolerate them.

Risk assessment is a complex area that requires the application of all the principles of toxicology. It is often divided into four somewhat overlapping areas:

(1) hazard identification
(2) dose–response assessment
(3) exposure assessment
(4) risk characterization.

Hazard identification is the process of collecting and evaluating information on the effects of an agent on animal or human health and well-being. In most cases, this involves a careful assessment of the adverse effects and what is the most sensitive population. The dose–response assessment involves evaluation of the relationship between dose and adverse effect. Typically, an effort is made to determine the lowest dose or exposure at which an effect is observed. A comparison is often made between animal data and any human data that might be available. Next is exposure assessment, in which an evaluation of the likely exposure to any given population is assessed. Important parameters include the dose, duration, frequency, and route of exposure. The final step is risk characterization, in which all the above information is synthesized and a judgment made on what is an acceptable level of human exposure. In the simplest terms, risk is the product of two factors: hazard and exposure (i.e. hazard × exposure = risk). In real risk assessments, all hazards may not be known and exposure is often difficult to quantify precisely. As a result, the calculated risk may not accurately reflect the real risk. The accuracy of a risk assessment is no better than the data and assumptions upon which it is based.

Risk management is the political or social process of deciding how the benefits balance the associated risks. Risk management is also concerned with how the public perceives risk and how we judge and perform our own risk assessments. An example of risk management was the decision to remove lead from gasoline. After a great deal of research it was demonstrated that low levels of lead exposure are harmful to the developing nervous system. It was then determined that this benefit of removing lead from gasoline was greater than the costs. A program was then developed to phase out lead from gasoline gradually in line with the engines of new cars not requiring lead and the replacement of old cars.

## 2.9 Summary

The principles of toxicology are summarized as follows: dose–response, risk = hazard × exposure and individual sensitivity. Many of us have an excellent intuitive sense of the principles of toxicology from experience with caffeine, alcohol, or other drug exposures. These experiences form a foundation upon which to build a formal understanding of toxicology that is applicable to many situations. We make many personal decisions based on dose–response and risk consideration. Around our home we must decide which cleaning products to use or whether to apply pesticides to our lawn or garden. As citizens we are also confronted with many broader concerns about environmental exposures. How much do we invest to limit the spread of environmental contaminants? Should coal-fired power generating facilities be required to invest in more sophisticated smoke stack scrubbers to remove mercury? On what basis do we make this decision? Advances in the toxicological sciences along with general advances in the biological sciences provide new knowledge and understanding upon which to make these and other decisions. And finally, I hope that beyond the principles of toxicology you will find that toxicology is both fun and informative.

## 2.10 Slide Presentation

■   Principles of Toxicology presentation material. Online. Available HTTP: <http://www.crcpress.com/e_products/> and follow the links to downloads and then the catalog number TF1691.
Web site contains presentation material related to the principles of toxicology.

# Part 1

# Toxic agents

# Chapter 3

# Alcohol

## Contents

### 3.1 Dossier

**Name:** Ethyl alcohol ($CH_3$-$CH_2$-OH)
**Use:** solvent, commonly found in beverages
**Source:** home, industry, stores, and alcoholic beverages
**Recommended daily intake:** none (not essential)
**Absorption:** readily absorbed by intestine, food will delay absorption
**Sensitive individuals:** fetus (fetal alcohol syndrome – FAS)
**Toxicity/symptoms:** developing nervous system very sensitive to low levels of exposure; children – lowered IQ, learning and behavioral problems; adults – memory loss, inebriation, liver disease, cancer

> **Regulatory facts:** government agencies recommend women do not consume alcohol during pregnancy; blood alcohol regulated by local governments when operating a motor vehicle
> **General facts:** long history of use, consumed worldwide, 1–3 infants per 1000 affected by FAS worldwide
> **Environmental:** voluntarily consumed
> **Recommendations:** do not consume alcohol during pregnancy, otherwise, limit consumption and do not drive a motor vehicle after drinking

Alcohol is the number one drug of choice among our nation's youth. Yet the seriousness of this issue does not register with the general public or policymakers.
Enoch Gordis, M.D. Director, National Institute on Alcohol Abuse and Alcoholism.

## 3.2 Case studies

### 3.2.1 Fetal alcohol syndrome

Despite its long history of use, the effects of alcohol on the developing fetus were not recognized until the early 1970s. Fetal alcohol syndrome (FAS) is the result of maternal consumption of alcohol during pregnancy and is one of the leading causes of learning disabilities and physical growth deficiency. FAS is identified by characteristic changes in facial features particularly around the mouth and eyes. A milder form without the facial deformities, but with associated learning disabilities and central nervous system (CNS) dysfunction, is called fetal alcohol effect (FAE) or alcohol-related neurodevelopmental disorder (ARND). In the US, it is estimated that between 4,000 and 12,000 infants suffer from FAS and 36,000 children have milder forms of alcohol related disabilities. Worldwide, as many as three infants per 1000 births have FAS, and an unknown number are afflicted with milder forms of disability related to maternal alcohol consumption. The obvious effects of alcohol on the infant clearly illustrate the sensitivity of the developing fetus to the chemical exposure. The tragedy is twofold:

(1) the effects of alcohol on the fetus are totally preventable
(2) the effects last a lifetime, robbing the individual of their full genetic potential.

### 3.2.2 Alcohol and the liver

Alcohol has a range of effects: for some, desirable acute effects; unwanted effects on the developing fetus; and with long-term consumption, effects on the liver and other organs. In the US, over 2 million people experience alcohol related liver disease. Effects on the liver are dose related; the more you consume the greater the effects. Early on there is an accumulation of fat in the liver as a result of the metabolism of alcohol. Some heavy drinkers develop an inflammation (alcoholic hepatitis) of the liver. Metabolites of alcohol, produced by the liver, are toxic to the liver cells.

As the process continues, the liver becomes less functional and a fibrosis process starts that can lead to cirrhosis or scarring of the liver. Continued drinking can result in death, but if the drinking stops, function of the liver can improve although the damage is irreversible.

### 3.3 Introduction and history

'T is not the drinking that is to be blamed, but the excess.
John Selden (1584–1654) In "Table Talk" 1689

Viewed through the lens of toxicology, alcoholic beverages provide a fascinating window into our relationship with a substance that many of us consume because of its intoxicating properties. Our love/hate relationship with alcoholic beverages began over 10,000 years ago with the accidental fermentation of beer. The production of wine soon followed and cultivation of vineyards is documented by about 3000 BC. The ancient ruler of Babylon, Hammurabi, commented on the purchase and sale of wine in rules set down in 2000 BC. The Greek god of wine, Dionysus, taught the cultivation of vines and frolic in 1500 BC. The combination of lead and wine may have helped bring down the Roman Empire. The use of alcoholic beverages was constantly being shaped by the technology of the era and various attempts by society to regulate its consumption. But despite our great familiarity with alcohol, it was not until the late 1960s that we realized that alcohol consumption during pregnancy severely affects the developing infant with no harm to the mother.

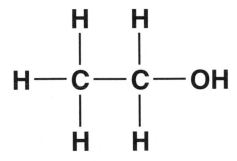

Whiskey – water of life (Gaelic *uisge beatha*) – Alcohol was once thought to be a cure for many illnesses including the common cold.

The word alcohol comes from the Arabic *al-kuhul*, originally referring to a white powder of antimony used as eye make-up. Alchemists of the 16th century began referring to alcohol as the essence from distillation, thus the essences of wine. It was not until the middle of the 18th century that alcohol took on its current meaning of the intoxicating ingredient of many common beverages.

Alcohols are a large class of compounds characterized by having an OH (oxygen and hydrogen) group attached to a carbon atom. The simplest alcohol is methanol or wood alcohol ($CH_3$-OH). Methanol is highly toxic and an undesirable contaminant of an alcoholic beverage. Ethyl alcohol, the intoxicating alcohol of many beverages, is $CH_3$-$CH_2$-OH.

Fermentation – sugar to alcohol and carbon dioxide

$$C_6H_{12}O_6 \rightarrow 2C_2H_5OH + 2CO_2$$

The accidental fermentation of grain probably produced the first beer. Fermentation occurs when microorganisms such as yeast, fungi, or bacteria break down complex molecules to produce energy in the absence of oxygen. Most often, fermentation produces unpleasant acids, but yogurt, cheese, sauerkraut, and black tea depend on fermentation. During fermentation certain strains of yeast produce ethyl alcohol and carbon dioxide in their quest for energy from available sugars. Below is a list of common fermentation starting points and the end products either as a direct result of fermentation of from further distillation.

- Cereal grains → beers and whiskeys
- Honey → mead
- Grapes → wine and brandy
- Root vegetables → vodka
- Sugar cane → rum

> Beer fact – The dark porter beers were developed in London, England in 1722 to nourish potters and heavy laborers.
>
> An Irish brewer named Guinness refined this process in the late 1700s to produce a beer that still bears his name.

## 3.4 Biological properties

Alcohol is an excellent and widely used solvent, appearing in many products from gasoline to drugs, and of course in common alcoholic beverages. Industrially it is produced by chemical reactions using acetaldehyde or petroleum byproducts and more recently from biomass, primarily corn. In the United States, ethanol production for use in fuel has grown from 175 million gallons in 1980 to over 1.4 billion gallons in 1998 (1 US gallon is equivalent to 3.79 liters).

Alcohol, or more precisely ethanol, is readily absorbed from the stomach and the intestine. Elapsed time from the last drink of alcohol to the highest blood level is about 30 minutes. As direct experience bears out, alcohol absorption is slowed by the presence of food in the stomach; however, once it reaches the small intestine, however, alcohol absorption is rapid. Alcohol can also be absorbed by the lungs and can be a significant industrial hazard.

Most of the alcohol distributes into body water, but like most solvents and anesthetics some distributes into fat. It is excreted in the urine and breath, hence the utility of taking breath samples to evaluate alcohol exposure. The majority of alcohol is metabolized in the liver. Alcohol dehydrogenase (ADH) metabolizes alcohol to acetaldehyde. Acetaldehyde is toxic, with elevated levels causing flushing, headache, nausea, and vomiting. Acetaldehyde is in turn quickly metabolized to the less toxic acetate by acetaldehyde dehydrogenase (ALDH) (Figure 3.1).

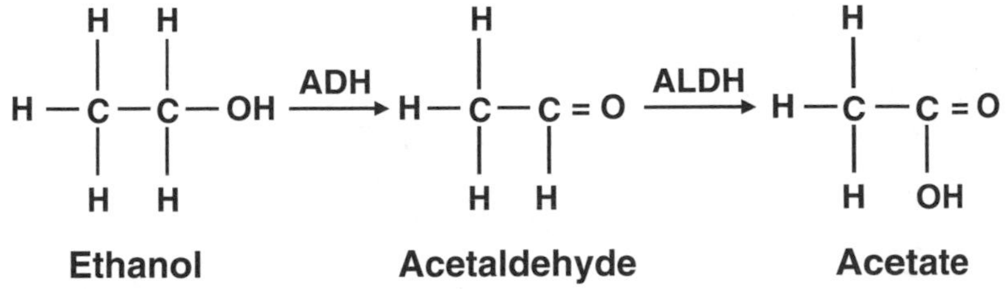

**Figure 3.1.** Metabolism of alcohol.

Humans have varying amounts and types of ALDH and this affects the metabolism of the toxic acetaldehyde. Approximately 50% of Asians have a single base change in a gene that encodes for ALDH, which results in an inactive form of ALDH. For a person with inactive ALDH, alcohol consumption can be very unpleasant. Antabuse (disulfiram), a drug prescribed to discourage alcohol consumption, blocks ALDH causing blood levels of acetaldehyde to rise and the subsequent toxic side effects discourage continued alcohol consumption. Disulfiram was a chemical originally used in the rubber industry. Workers inadvertently exposed to disulfiram accidentally discovered its effects when they became sick after drinking alcoholic beverages.

The metabolism of most drugs or chemicals is proportional to the concentration in the blood, which allows a half-life to be calculated. Ethanol is different; its metabolism is relatively constant over time and does not increase with rising blood ethanol concentrations. Metabolism is proportional to body weight; thus the bigger you are, the higher the rate of ethanol metabolism, but on average ethanol is metabolized at a rate of 120 mg/kg per hour or about 1 oz (30 ml) in 3 hours.

Ethanol is readily measured in the blood and reported as milligrams per milliliter (mg per ml) of blood. Laws regulating drinking and driving identify a specific blood alcohol concentration (BAC) as unacceptable when operating a motor vehicle. Currently most states set 0.08 or 0.1, which is equivalent to 80 mg/100 ml or 80 mg/dl of blood. Alcohol content of exhaled breath is about 0.05% of the BAC.

Another factor in determining blood alcohol concentrations and thus the effects of alcohol is gender. Drink for drink, a female will have a higher BAC than a male. First, women tend to be smaller, so by body weight they receive a higher dose of alcohol. Second, women metabolize less alcohol in the intestine than men, which results in greater absorption of alcohol and hence higher BAC. Finally, women have a greater proportion of body fat, which results in a lower volume of fluid by weight. An average male of medium weight (160–180 pounds) must consume 4 drinks in an hour to reach a BAC of 0.08, whereas an average female weighing 130 to 140 pounds would require only 3 drinks within one hour.

The mechanisms of action of the effects of alcohol on the nervous system remain unclear. For some time, researchers thought that the depressant effects of alcohol, like other anesthetic agents, were caused by dissolving into the cell lipid membranes and disrupting the function of various proteins. More recently, researchers have focused on specific receptors such as glutamate (excitatory) and GABA (inhibitory). Despite intensive research, the mechanism of effect of alcohol on the fetus is unknown.

## 3.5 Health effects

By any measure, alcohol has an enormous impact on our society: it contributes to 100,000 deaths and costs $166 billion in the US alone. The toxic effects of alcohol have resulted in many efforts and laws to control and regulate its consumption. While alcohol affects the individual consumer, there are two areas of particular concern:

(1)  the effects of alcohol on the developing infant from maternal alcohol consumption
(2)  the death and injury caused by driving motor vehicles following drinking.

The health effects of alcohol section is divided into children and adults to emphasize the sensitivity of fetal exposure to alcohol during pregnancy.

Before starting, it is necessary to define what a drink means. This is not as straightforward as it might seem given the wide range of beverages that contain varying amounts of alcohol. The common definition of a drink is a beverage that contains 0.5 oz or 15 ml of ethanol.

---

**A drink is defined as 0.5 oz (15 ml) of ethanol:**

One 12-oz (360 ml) bottle of beer
One 5-oz (150 ml) glass of wine
1.5 oz (45 ml) of 80-proof distilled spirits

The percent ethanol in any beverage will vary. For example, wine can range from 8 to 15%.

---

### 3.5.1 Children

Despite alcohol's long history of use, the association of adverse effects of maternal alcohol consumption on the developing fetus were first described in 1968 by French researchers at the University of Nantes. In 1972, the cluster of effects was further described and named fetal alcohol syndrome (FAS) by researchers at the University of Washington, Seattle, WA, US. FAS is characterized by physical and facial abnormalities (Figure 3.2), slow growth, CNS dysfunction, and other disabilities. The brain damage can be severe, leaving the child with serious learning and functional disabilities that last a lifetime. Fetal alcohol effect (FAE) designates children born with learning or memory disabilities but without the characteristic physical deformities. Alcohol consumption during pregnancy also causes an increase in stillbirths and spontaneous abortions. Alcohol consumption during pregnancy results in the largest number of preventable mental disabilities in the world.

In 1981 the US Surgeon General first advised that women should not drink alcoholic beverages during pregnancy because of the risks to the infant. In 1989 warning labels were mandated on all alcoholic beverages sold in the United States, and since 1990 the US government has clearly stated that women who are pregnant or planning to become pregnant should not drink alcohol.

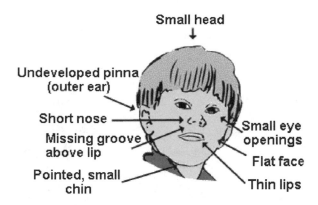

**Figure 3.2.** Effects of *in utero* alcohol exposure.

It is difficult to determine exactly how many young children and subsequent adults are handicapped by fetal exposure to alcohol because the diagnosis of less severe forms of fetal alcohol effects is imprecise. Worldwide, alcohol consumption affects between 1 and 3 out of 1000 infants. In the United States, 4000 to 12,000 infants per year are born with FAS and three times as many with more minor effects. A 1998 study in the United States found that over 50% of women drank alcohol during pregnancy. An additional concern is that a woman is often not aware of being pregnant during the first few weeks of pregnancy.

The consequences of maternal alcohol consumption are tragic and last a lifetime for the exposed infant. In 1989, Michael Dorris described the life of his adopted son Able as that of a drowning man, one "conceived in an ethanol bath" unable to find the shore.

### 3.5.2 Adults

Alcohol, a toxic solvent, flows freely in our society. Because it is heavily advertised, easy to make, easier to purchase, and widely consumed across all ages because of its neuroactive properties, we struggle to address a wide range of health consequences of alcohol consumption. In the United States the legal drinking age is 21 years, but consumption of alcoholic beverages often starts much earlier. In Europe and other parts of the world the legal drinking age is generally 18 and sometimes 16 years of age. The health effects of alcohol are related to its acute effects on the nervous system and longer-term effects from chronic consumption.

The main acute effect is inebriation, which in turn spawns violence, spousal and child abuse, crime, motor vehicle accidents, workplace and home accidents, drowning, suicide, and accidental death. The chronic effects include alcoholism, liver disease, various forms of cancer, brain disorders, cardiovascular disease and other organ system effects, absence from or loss of work, family dysfunction, and malnutrition.

The acute effects of alcohol consumption are associated with mild nervous system effects such as relaxation and a lessening of inhibitions that many people find desirable. Additional consumption results in sleepiness and motor and reaction time effects such as those used in operating a motor vehicle. Continued consumption can result in drunkenness, which is often associated with uncontrolled mood swings and emotional response and sometimes violence. Excessive consumption or very rapid consumption of large quantities of alcohol can result in respiratory depression, coma, and possibly death. Vasodilation also occurs, especially in vessels near the skin, which gives an impression of warmth. Contrary to popular belief, sexual function is decreased for both men and women.

Chronic consumption of alcohol can result in a tolerance to its overt effects but it still affects functional ability, such as that required to drive a vehicle. Tolerance can develop to such an extent that an individual can have very high alcohol levels (300 to 400 mg/dl) and still not appear to be affected. However, the ability to tolerate high blood alcohol levels does not change the level necessary to produce death.

---

Alcohol withdrawal effects:

- Tremor
- Nausea
- Irritability
- Agitation
- Tachycardia
- Hypertension
- Seizures
- Hallucinations

---

Chronic excessive consumption of alcohol can result in physical dependence or alcoholism. There is often a steady progress in the need to drink, so that the person starts drinking early in the day to maintain blood alcohol levels and avoid withdrawal effects. Alcoholism often results in a variety of organ system effects, some of which are related to accompanying malnutrition. Treatment for alcoholism must address the withdrawal effects as well as associated vitamin deficiencies associated with malnutrition.

Alcohol affects a range of organs but clearly the most common effects are associated with liver disease. Initially there is accumulation of fat in the liver. Cellular damage appears to be associated with increased levels of acetaldehyde. This in turn results in a scarring or hardening of the liver called cirrhosis. All these changes to the liver will result in decreased ability to metabolize alcohol as well as other drugs, or will even enhance the toxicity of some drugs, for example acetaminophen (paracetamol).

Alcohol is classified as an agent "known to be a human carcinogen" for causing cancer of the mouth, oral cavity, and esophagus. Alcohol is also associated with a general increase in cancer of other organs such as the liver and interacts synergistically with smoking, putting smokers at a greater risk for developing cancer. There is increasing evidence that alcohol consumption by women increases the risk for breast cancer.

## 3.6 Reducing exposure

Reducing exposure is easy in concept but sometimes more difficult in practice: just don't drink alcoholic beverages or drink less. Most importantly, women who are planning on becoming pregnant or are pregnant should not consume alcohol. Men need to support and encourage this position. For many that consume alcohol, it is important to learn how to manage exposure. Food consumption slows alcohol absorption, so eat while drinking so as not to consume alcohol on an empty stomach. There is a great amount of variability in the percent of alcohol in drinks. It is a good practice to consume less of drinks with high alcohol content.

## 3.7 Regulatory standards

- 1981 – US Surgeon General first advised that women should not drink alcoholic beverages during pregnancy.
- 1988 – US requires warning labels on all alcoholic beverages sold in the United States.
- 1990 – US Dietary Guidelines state that women who are pregnant or planning to become pregnant should not drink alcohol.
- 1998 – 19 states require the posting of alcohol health warning signs where alcoholic beverages are sold.

## 3.8 Recommendation and conclusions

Alcohol is a very toxic agent causing enormous suffering. The most tragic effects occur when a woman consumes alcohol during pregnancy, producing irreversible harm to the developing fetus. The consumption of alcohol during pregnancy is the single greatest cause of preventable birth defects, and learning and performance disabilities. Needless to say, alcohol is associated with motor vehicle accidents and a range of other detrimental effects. Over $1 billion is spent every year advertising the consumption of this drug.

## 3.9 More information and references

### 3.9.1 Slide presentation

- A Small Dose of Alcohol presentation material. Online. Available HTTP: <http://www.crcpress.com/e_products/> and follow the links to downloads and then the catalog number TF1691.
  Web site contains presentation material related to the toxicity of alcohol.

### 3.9.2 European, Asian, and international agencies

- England – Department of Health (DOH) Alcohol Misuse Information. Online. Available HTTP: <http://www.doh.gov.uk/alcohol/index.htm> (accessed: 1 April 2003).
  The DOH provides extensive information on the health effects of alcohol.

- Nordic Council for Alcohol and Drug Research (NAD). Online. Available HTTP: <http://www.kaapeli.fi/nad/> (accessed: 2 April 2003).
- International Council on Alcohol and Addictions (ICAA). Online. Available HTTP: <http://www.icaa.de/> (accessed: 2 April 2003).
  "ICAA is a non-governmental organization in consultative status (Category Special) with the Economic and Social Council of the United Nations and in official relations with the World Health Organization."

### 3.9.3 North American agencies

- Health Canada – Fetal Alcohol Syndrome and Fetal Alcohol Effect. Online. Available HTTP: <http://www.hc-sc.gc.ca/fnihb/cp/fas_fae/index.htm> (accessed: 2 April 2003).
  This site provides tool to reduce and manage the effects of fetal exposure to alcohol.
- US National Institute on Alcohol Abuse and Alcoholism (NIAAA). Online. Available HTTP: <http://www.niaaa.nih.gov/> (accessed: 2 April 2003).
  "The NIAAA supports and conducts biomedical and behavioral research on the causes, consequences, treatment, and prevention of alcoholism and alcohol-related problems."
- Alcohol – Center for the Evaluation of Risks to Human Reproduction (CERHR) – The National Toxicology Program. Online. Available HTTP: <http://cerhr.niehs.nih.gov/genpub/topics/alcohol2-ccae.html> (accessed: 5 April 2003).
  CERHR alcohol web site has information for parents about the effects of alcohol on reproduction and development.
- US National Clearinghouse for Alcohol and Drug Information (NCADI). Online. Available HTTP: <http://www.health.org/> (accessed: 2 April 2003).
  "NCADI is the world's largest resource for current information and materials concerning substance abuse."
- US Center for Substance Abuse Prevention (CSAP). Online. Available HTTP: <http://prevention.samhsa.gov/> (accessed: 2 April 2003).
  "The CSAP mission is to decrease substance use and abuse by bringing effective prevention to every community."

### 3.9.4 Non-government organizations

- Alcoholics Anonymous (AA). Online. Available HTTP: <http://www.aa.org/> (accessed: 2 April 2003).
  An international organization dedicated to helping people with alcohol consumptions concerns.
- Center for Science in the Public Interest (CSPI). Online. Available HTTP: <http://www.cspinet.org/> (accessed: 2 April 2003).
  "CSPI is an advocate for nutrition and health, food safety, alcohol policy, and sound science."
- Mothers Against Drunk Driving (MADD). Online. Available HTTP: <http://www.madd.org/> (accessed: 2 April 2003).

"MADD's mission is to stop drunk driving, support the victims of this violent crime, and prevent underage drinking."

- National Council on Alcoholism and Drug Dependence, Inc. (NCADD). Online. Available HTTP: <http://www.ncadd.org/> (accessed: 2 April 2003). NCADD provides education, information, help and hope to the public and advocates prevention, intervention, and treatment.

- Rutgers Center of Alcohol Studies (CAS). Online. Available HTTP: <http://www.rci.rutgers.edu/~cas2/> (accessed: 2 April 2003).
  The Center of Alcohol Studies (CAS) is a multidisciplinary institute dedicated to acquisition and dissemination of knowledge on psychoactive substance use and related phenomena with primary emphasis on alcohol use and consequences.

- FAS Bookshelf, Inc. Online. Available HTTP: <http://www.fasbookshelf.com/index.html> (accessed: 2 April 2003).
  Web site devoted to providing resources on fetal alcohol syndrome.

- National Organization on Fetal Alcohol Syndrome. Online. Available HTTP: <http://www.nofas.org/> (accessed: 2 April 2003).
  "NOFAS is a nonprofit organization founded in 1990 dedicated to eliminating birth defects caused by alcohol consumption during pregnancy and improving the quality of life for those individuals and families affected."

- The Alcohol and Temperance History Group (ATHG). Online. Available HTTP: <http://www.athg.org/> (accessed: 2 April 2003).
  "ATHG was founded in 1979 to foster the exchange of ideas among scholars of all disciplines who are interested in any aspect of past alcohol use, abuse, production, and control within given societies or countries."

### 3.9.5 References

- Alcohol and Health, 10th Special Report to the US Congress. Highlights from Current Research. Health and Human Services, June 2000.

- *Fetal Alcohol Syndrome – Diagnosis, Epidemiology, Prevention, and Treatment*, Kathleen Stratton, Cynthia Howe, and Frederick C. Battaglia, eds; Committee to Study Fetal Alcohol Syndrome, Institute of Medicine, Washington, DC, 1996. Web Access: http://www.nap.edu/catalog/4991.html?se_side

- *Global Status Report: Alcohol and Young People*, by David H. Jernigan. World Health Organization, 2001. Access: http://www.who.int/en/, (use search) Date: September 15, 2002.

# Chapter 4

# Caffeine

## Contents

- Dossier
- Case studies
- Introduction and history
- Biological properties
- Health effects
- Reducing exposure
- Regulatory standards
- Recommendation and conclusions
- More information and references

## 4.1 Dossier

**Name:** caffeine (1,3,7-trimethylxanthine)

**Use:** most widely used stimulant in the world

**Source:** coffee, tea, cola and other soft drinks, chocolate

**Recommended daily intake:** the US Food and Drug Administration (FDA) advised pregnant women to "avoid caffeine-containing foods and drugs, if possible, or consume them only sparingly"

**Absorption:** rapid following oral consumption

**Sensitive individuals:** fetus, children, some adults

**Toxicity/symptoms:** high dose – agitation, tremors; withdrawal – headache

**Regulatory facts:** GRAS (generally recognized as safe)

**General facts:** long history of use
  Related xanthines – theobromine (3,7-dimethylxanthin) and theophylline (1,3-dimethylxanthine)
**Environmental:** contaminates sewage discharge

## Caffeine industry

The coffee and cola industries owe their wealth to the physiological properties of the drug caffeine.

S. G. Gilbert (2001)

## Coffee

Black as hell, strong as death, sweet as love.

Turkish proverb

Often coffee drinkers, finding the drug to be unpleasant, turn to other narcotics, of which opium and alcohol are most common.

*Morphinism and Narcomanias from Other Drugs* (1902) by
T. D. Crothers, M.D.

Coffee, which makes the politician wise,
And see through all things with his half-shut eyes.

Alexander Pope (1688–1744), English satirical poet.
*Rape of the Lock,* cto. 3 (1712).

The morning cup of coffee has an exhilaration about it which the cheering influence of the afternoon or evening cup of tea cannot be expected to reproduce.

Oliver Wendell Holmes Sr. (1809–94), US writer, physician.
*Over the Teacups,* ch. 1 (1891).

## Tea

Is there no Latin word for Tea? Upon my soul, if I had known that I would have let the vulgar stuff alone.

Hilaire Belloc (1870–1953), British author.
*On Nothing,* "On Tea" (1908).

It has been well said that tea is suggestive of a thousand wants, from which spring the decencies and luxuries of civilization.

Agnes Repplier (1858–1950), US author, social critic.
*To Think of Tea!* ch. 2 (1932).

> Tea, though ridiculed by those who are naturally coarse in their nervous sensibilities . . . will always be the favorite beverage of the intellectual.
>
> Thomas De Quincey (1785–1859), English author.
> *Confessions of an English Opium-Eater*,
> "The Pleasures of Opium" (1822).

## 4.2 Case studies

### 4.2.1 The individual

With a drug that is as commonly consumed and easily available as caffeine, the very best case study is yourself, your family, or your friends. Ask the following questions and carefully consider the implications of these answers. Have you ever drunk too much caffeine? If so, how did you know you had too much? If the answer to the first question is yes, then you are on your way to becoming a toxicologist. If you have felt the jitters or agitation of too much caffeine, then you have experienced the nervous system effects that can be called a form of neurotoxicology and you are on your way to becoming a neurotoxicologist.

An additional question related to the nervous system effects of caffeine is what happens when you stop drinking caffeine? Do you get a headache? If the answer is yes then you are dependent on the drug caffeine. Some of your caffeine consumption is driven by a desire to avoid a caffeine-induced headache.

How many hours elapse before you reach for that second cup of coffee? Many of us have learned by practice that when our blood caffeine levels decline too far, we need to boost them back up with a second cup of coffee, tea, or a can of soft drink.

The above factors make caffeine the most widely consumed stimulant drug in the world. The stimulant and other basic biological properties of caffeine make it an almost ideal drug for many large corporations and small businesses to make large amounts of money.

### 4.2.2 The society

The study of caffeine is a window into our culture and society. Why do so many people consume caffeine and what does that say about our drug consumption? What are the basic biological properties that make caffeine the most widely consumed stimulant in the world and allow a number of international corporations to make vast sums of money?

Many people start consuming caffeine at an early age. It is not uncommon for schools to have soft drink machines and even coffee stands at and certainly near schools. Middle and high school students are well aware of the stimulant properties of caffeine. Is it appropriate to have soft drink machines in schools, which encourages caffeine consumption?

## 4.3 Introduction and history

> If Christianity is wine, and Islam coffee, Buddhism is most certainly tea.
>
> Alan Watts, *The Way of Zen*, 1957

Caffeine, a naturally occurring chemical found in a number of plants, has a long and illustrious history and continues to have an enormous impact on our society. It has gone from being vilified and compared to alcohol and nicotine to become the most widely accepted and consumed neuroactive drug in the world. Caffeine is available in a wide range of products with no regulations on its sale or use. Caffeine, even more than alcohol and nicotine, demonstrates the human interest and capacity to consume drugs that affect our nervous system.

In this chapter we will explore why we so readily consume caffeine. There are sound physiological reasons why so many companies make so much money from caffeine. The economics are staggering. Coffee alone is one of the largest cash crops in the world. It is estimated that in 1998/1999 coffee production was greater that 6 billion kilograms (more that 12 billion pounds), which would translate into over a trillion cups of coffee and literally tons of caffeine. This does not even take into consideration the caffeine consumed from cola beverages, tea, and chocolate. Our brains and our wallets are hooked on caffeine.

Historically, caffeine has played an important role in trade and politics and even now the export of coffee is an extremely important part of world trade for many countries. The health effects of caffeine have been the subject of numerous scientific inquiries, many scientific papers and conferences, and many books and articles. Perhaps the best book to combine both historical and health aspects of caffeine is *The World of Caffeine – The Science and Culture of the World's Most Popular Drug* by Bennett Alan Weinberg and Bonnie K. Bealer, published in 2001. This book gives a wonderful account of the interaction of caffeine and society from its ancient roots to present times, as well as a look at the health effects. A book devoted almost entirely to the health effects of caffeine is *Caffeine and Health* by Jack E. James, published in 1991. There is no lack of information on caffeine.

Given the many plants that contain caffeine, some have speculated that even Stone Age humans chewed the leaves and fruit of caffeine-producing plants to enjoy its stimulant properties. Although this early consumption is speculative, it is clear that caffeine consumption has been with us for a long time.

Tea appears to be the most ancient of caffeine drinks. The first documented use is in China by its first great emperor, Shen Nung, in about 2700 BC. Throughout Chinese history there are many references to tea and its many benefits. The earliest written record of tea consumption is from a Chinese document from 350 BC. Tea became popular with Buddhist monks to keep them awake during long hours of meditation. Despite the association of tea with China, some believe that tea was actually introduced into China from Northern India. In the 5th century, tea was an important aspect of trade on the Silk Road to China. About AD 800 tea was introduced to Japan. In Japan the consumption of tea, more specifically a green powdered tea, evolved into an elaborate ceremony that is still practiced today. The Dutch brought tea to Europe in 1610, and the Americans revolted over taxes on tea in 1773. A few years later, England sent the first opium to China in payment for tea, which ultimately resulted in the Opium Wars and England's control of Hong Kong. Tea bags were accidentally invented in 1908. In more recent times, we are treated to a great many fragrant varieties of tea from around the world.

Coffee's history is equally rich. According to the legends, in about AD 850, an Ethiopian goatherd (or shepherd depending on your source) noticed that his goats seemed more alert after consuming wild berries. Wishing to increase his own performance, he tried the berries himself, constituting the first occupational consumption of coffee. The cultivation of coffee shrubs and roasting of coffee beans was developed by 1100. Four hundred years later, Mecca, Cairo, and Constantinople were the sites of the first coffee shops. Coffee came to Europe in the 1600s and quickly spread to the Americas. By the 1700s there were coffee shops throughout Europe, and coffee was fast becoming part of the culture. Coffee trees were introduced into the Americas in 1723. The first espresso machines were made in France in the early 1800s, and the early 1900s saw the introduction of instant coffee. In 1971, the first Starbuck's coffee shop was opened in Seattle, Washington and 30 years later there are thousands of Starbucks around the world. In many parts of the world, coffee shops are an important gathering place for discussion and relaxation, an integral aspect of people's culture. In this respect, the United States is just catching up to the rest of the world.

Chocolate provides much less caffeine than tea or coffee, but people all over the world consume it not so much for the caffeine but for the taste. Archeological evidence indicates that the Olmec people of Mexico harvested the cacao bean to make a drink in 400 BC or perhaps earlier. By AD 250, the Mayans of Mexico were cultivating the cacao tree. The Aztec people used the cacao bean as currency and equated it to a drink from the Gods. The scientific name for the cacao bean tree is *Theobroma cacao*. *Theobroma* is Greek for "Food of the Gods". Theobromine, the primary caffeine-like compound found in chocolate, also derives its name from *theobroma*. The Spanish explorer Hernando Cortés brought cocoa to Spain in 1528, where it was kept secret from the rest of Europe until 1600 when it quickly became very popular, so popular that the Pope had to declare that chocolate drink did not break a fast. The first English chocolate houses opened up in 1657. In 1828, shortly after the invention of the first espresso machine, the screw press for extracting cocoa butter from the beans was invented in Holland. Chocolate as a solid was invented in the 1840s and soon it was a staple of solders at war and just about everyone else.

A glance at Tables 4.1 and 4.2 illustrates how caffeine cuts across society, trade, politics, and industry to become the drug of choice for billions of people. The amount of caffeine in a particular product, as well as the amount consumed, can vary enormously. The amount of caffeine in a cup of coffee varies with the type of bean, the roasting, and the type of brewing method employed. The cup size adds another variable. Tea actually has a higher concentration of caffeine than coffee, but the extraction of the caffeine from coffee is more efficient than that of tea. If you want more caffeine in your tea, however, you only need to brew it for a longer period of time. By weight, cocoa has the least amount of caffeine, but it also has the

### Table 4.1 Common products and caffeine concentration

| Product | Caffeine (mg) | Size |
|---|---|---|
| Coffee | 50–150 | Cup about 8 ounces or 225 ml |
| Tea | 20–100 | Cup about 8 ounces or 225 ml |
| Cola drink | 20–100 | 8 ounce or 225 ml |
| Chocolate (cocoa) | 1–35 | One ounce or 28 grams |

**Table 4.2 History of caffeine consumption (T = tea, Co = coffee, Ch = chocolate)**

| Date | Type | Event |
|---|---|---|
| 3000 BC | T | Tea discovered in China or introduced from India |
| 350 BC | T | First written description of tea drinking in China |
| 400 BC | Ch | Olmec people of Mexico made chocolate drinks |
| AD 250 | Ch | Mayans of Mexico were cultivating cocoa crops |
| 450 | T | Turkish traders bargain for tea and the Silk Road is born |
| 800 | T | Tea introduced to Japan |
| 850 (about) | Co | Coffee beans discovered – The fable says that an Ethiopian goatherder or sheepherder noticed that the goats were more alert after eating the wild berries. He then sampled this new delicacy |
| 1100 (about) | Co | First cultivation of coffee shrubs and roasting of coffee beans |
| 1450 | T | Japanese tea ceremony created and popularized |
| 1475 | Co | Constantinople – the world's first coffee house |
| 1528 | Ch | Cocoa was brought to Spain by Hernando Cortés |
| 1600s | Co | Coffee enters Europe and moves quickly to the Americas |
| 1600s | Ch | Chocolate drinks introduced into Europe |
| 1610 | T | Dutch bring tea to Europe |
| 1657 | Ch | First English chocolate houses open |
| 1700s | Co | Coffee house open throughout Europe |
| 1723 | Co | First coffee shrubs are introduced into the Americas |
| 1773 | T | Boston Tea party, rebellion against England's tea tax |
| 1776 | T | England sends first opium to China to help pay for tea |
| 1822 | Co | First espresso machine is created in France |
| 1828 | Ch | Screw press that extracted the cocoa butter from the beans invented in Holland |
| 1835 | T | First experimental tea plantations in Assam, India |
| 1840s | Ch | Chocolate as solid developed |
| 1908 | T | Tea bags invented in New York |
| 1938 | Co | First instant coffee invented by the Nestlé company |
| 1971 | Co | Starbucks opens its first location in Seattle, Washington's Pike Place Market |

structurally similar compound theobromine. Caffeine is added to many cola and other soft drink beverages. Some are known for their high caffeine concentration. It is now possible to buy water-based drinks fortified with caffeine. Over-the-counter pills of caffeine are available, and many analgesic medications contain caffeine as well, in part to alleviate the headache due to lack of caffeine.

## 4.4 Biological properties

Caffeine is a naturally occurring chemical manufactured by a number of plants in either the fruit – as in coffee bean, cola nuts, and cocoa beans – or the leaves – as in tea. The common use of caffeine-bearing substances throughout the world at the start of the 19th century coincided with a period of great discovery in the physical and chemical sciences. Caffeine was isolated from coffee beans in 1819 by Friedlieb Ferdinand Runge, a young German physician and chemist. Caffeine derives its name from the German *Kaffeine*, which is in turn from *Kaffee* or coffee. In 1827 the active ingredient in tea was isolated and called "thein", but was later found to be identical to the caffeine of coffee.

Purified, caffeine (Figure 4.1) is a white crystalline powder with a bitter taste. While caffeine is not particularly soluble in water, it is extracted from plant material with hot water. The longer the extraction period, the greater the amount of caffeine extracted. In plants, caffeine's purpose may be to discourage consumption by predators with its bitter taste and mild nervous system effects, but with humans it clearly has the opposite effect of encouraging consumption of the plant.

The chemical name of caffeine is 1,3,7-trimethylxanthine, and it is part of the purine family of derivatives of methylxanthines (Figure 4.2). Caffeine's basic chemical structure is similar to the purine structure found in DNA (see below). This similarity in structure generated speculation that caffeine may somehow cause

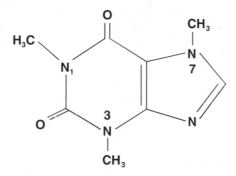

**Figure 4.1.** Caffeine (1,3,7-trimethylxanthine).

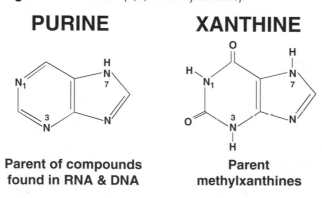

## PURINE

Parent of compounds
found in RNA & DNA

## XANTHINE

Parent
methylxanthines

**Figure 4.2.** Chemical structures of purine and xanthine.

cancer by interacting with DNA or RNA. Despite this similarity in structure, there is no indication that caffeine is mutagenic or causes cancer.

Closely related methylxanthines include theophylline (1,3-dimethylxanthine), theobromine (3,7-dimethylxanthine) and paraxanthine (1,7-dimethylxanthine). Theobromine is found primarily in chocolate. These derivatives of caffeine are important because they are pharmacologically active and also are the common metabolites of caffeine.

Caffeine is readily and completely absorbed from the intestine following oral ingestion. It distributes throughout body water, so that blood, urine, or breast milk will all have about the same concentration of caffeine. Metabolism varies between individuals, but on average the caffeine from a cup of coffee will produce peak blood caffeine levels in about 30 minutes. This peak level will drop by one-half in 4–5 hours, the so-called half-life. If you are a smoker, you will metabolize caffeine more quickly, usually with a half-life of about 3 hours. During pregnancy, the half-life of caffeine increases to 8–10 hours. The newborn child cannot metabolize caffeine and must rely solely on excretion of caffeine in the urine, which means the half-life of caffeine is measured in days not hours. Metabolism occurs primarily in the liver and starts with the removal of one or two of the methyl ($CH_3$) groups to make di- or monomethylxanthines, which are excreted in the liver. The relatively short half-life of caffeine is an important property of the drug and accounts for its repeated consumption. The half-life of theophylline is about twice that of caffeine.

Caffeine and the related dimethylxanthines have similar pharmacological or therapeutic effects and similar toxic effects. The primary actions include stimulation of the central nervous system, relaxation of bronchial muscles, mild cardiac muscle stimulation, and diuretic effects on the kidney.

There are a number of possible ways that caffeine can exert its effects, but the most probable action, particularly at concentrations from common consumption, is blockage of the adenosine receptor. Adenosine is a neurotransmitter that produces a calming effect. Caffeine blocks the receptors that are activated by adenosine, which results in stimulation (Figure 4.3). There is additional evidence that over time the cells of the nervous system respond to the blockage of adenosine receptors by increasing or up-regulating the number of adenosine receptors.

Caffeine and theophylline are more active on the central nervous system, while theobromine is much less active. Caffeine and theophylline also appear to stimulate the respiratory centers, making them useful in the treatment of infants who stop breathing for extended periods of time (sleep apnea), which can lead to sudden infant death.

Methylxanthines have a number of other effects, including effects on smooth muscles and the cardiovascular system. The most notable effect on smooth muscles is relaxing the bronchi of the lungs. Theophylline is prescribed to treat mild forms of asthma. While both caffeine and theophylline will relax the bronchial smooth muscles, theophylline is used therapeutically because of its longer half-life. This allows the drug to stay in the therapeutic range longer.

The caffeine naïve individual may notice some changes in heart rate following consumption of a strong cup of coffee. Most caffeine users have developed a tolerance to the cardiovascular effects, but these effects may occur if there is elevated consumption.

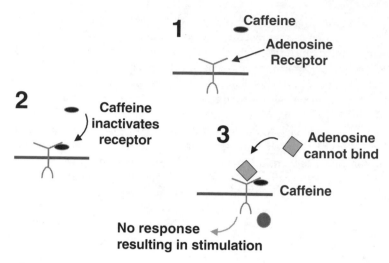

**Figure 4.3.** Mechanism of action of caffeine.

## 4.5 Health effects

Most people experience the stimulant effects of caffeine as an increase in alertness and energy and possibly an increase in concentration. What many like most is the ability to stay awake. Long-term consumption of caffeine does not seem to lessen the desirable effects of caffeine. In other words, long-term consumption of caffeine does not result in tolerance to the stimulatory effects. This is important for the caffeine industry because if we developed tolerance to this drug we would stop consuming it because of loss of effectiveness.

Another important aspect of caffeine is that repeated consumption does not change the metabolism of caffeine. From individual to individual, the half-life of caffeine in the blood (how fast it is removed) does not change with repeated use. If the half-life of caffeine decreased and the metabolism was faster, we would have to drink even more caffeine to maintain our blood caffeine levels.

The adverse effects of caffeine are a common experience to most caffeine consumers. Too much caffeine results in uncomfortable to adverse central nervous system effects, or neurotoxicity. The effects include restlessness, tension, and mild tremor or the jitters and may progress to feelings of anxiety and even fear. Regular caffeine users soon learn how to manage their caffeine consumption to maintain blood caffeine at a desirable level that produces mild stimulation without the uncomfortable neurotoxic effects. Fortunately, the half-life of caffeine is short, so that any undesirable effects soon decline. Many people also experience insomnia from caffeine consumption. Caffeine's effect on sleep varies from individual to individual. Some people can consume caffeine late in the evening and sleep well, but for other people consumption of caffeine late in the day affects sleep. It is important to understand your own individual response to caffeine.

Many people experience undesirable withdrawal effects when they stop consuming caffeine. The most prominent undesirable effect is a headache. Additional effects may include feelings of fatigue and irritability. Relief from symptoms usually occurs with resumption of caffeine consumption, a classic sign of drug dependence. Awareness of your individual potential to suffer from withdrawal effects of caffeine is important. This knowledge can often explain the onset of a headache when there is a sudden or unexpected cessation of caffeine consumption.

---

Chocolate contains theobromine, which can be toxic to dogs.

---

Most of the overt toxicity of the methyl xanthines, caffeine, theophylline and theobromine, is associated with the cardiovascular effects. Sensitive individuals may experience elevated or irregular heartbeats and elevated respiration. A good example of the cardiovascular effects of theobromine is evident when dogs consume chocolate. Milk chocolate contains about 45 mg/oz (150 mg/100 g) of theobromine and cooking chocolate about 400 mg/oz (1400 mg/100 g). The lethal effect of theobromine for dogs occurs at 100–150 mg/kg. In addition, the half-life of theobromine for a dog is about 17 hours. For a small dog it does not take much to produce serious toxic effects from the accidental consumption of chocolate. For example, 1 ounce (100 g) of cooking chocolate could be fatal for a dog weighing 22 pounds (10 kg). For humans the lethal effects of caffeine occur after consumption of between 5 and 10 grams, which on a mg/kg basis is similar to the 100–150 mg/kg of theobromine for dogs.

---

In 1980, the US Food and Drug Administration (FDA) advised pregnant women to "avoid caffeine-containing foods and drugs, if possible, or consume them only sparingly".

---

There are several good reasons to consider the potential for caffeine to affect the developing fetus. First, caffeine and its metabolites distribute throughout body water. This means that the fluid surrounding the fetus contains caffeine and its metabolites at levels similar to those in the mother's blood. The fetus is literally swimming in and breathing caffeine. Second, during the last two trimesters of pregnancy, maternal caffeine metabolism decreases. The half-life increases to about twice normal, or 8–10 hours. This means that after caffeine consumption the maternal blood caffeine levels and the infant's exposure will stay higher for a longer period of time. Third, caffeine clearly interacts with the nervous system by affecting the adenosine receptor. The consequences of having the fetal brain develop while being influenced by a drug that is blocking the adenosine receptor are not yet clear. There are some human and animal data indicating that high levels of caffeine may adversely affect the infant. The US FDA advises pregnant women to avoid or limit caffeine consumption in an effort to address these concerns.

People who drink caffeine have learned from experience how much to consume and thus to avoid the adverse behavioral effects of too much caffeine. Excessive consumption of caffeine is an almost perfect example of the fundamental dose–response principle of toxicology. A sudden reduction in caffeine consumption by the regular consumer can lead to the onset of headaches. It can be argued that many people are dependent on their caffeine consumption to maintain their body in a comfortable pain-free state. The mechanism responsible for the caffeine-induced headache is not understood. One possibility is that caffeine causes a small constriction of cerebral blood vessels. When caffeine consumption is stopped for an extended period of time these vessels enlarge causing a headache.

## 4.6 Reducing exposure

Many of us consume caffeine throughout our lives. Through experience we learn how much to consume to achieve the desired effects and avoid the undesirable ones. The first step in reducing exposure to any agent is being aware of the exposure and our response to it. It is simple to say that reducing exposure to caffeine only requires reduction in the consumption of caffeinated beverages. But in reality it is more complicated. For example, should there be easily available caffeinated products in high schools? What are the consequences of caffeine exposure to high school students?

## 4.7 Regulatory standards

The US Food and Drug Administration classifies caffeine as "generally recognized as safe" (GRAS). This designation means that there are sufficient data and history of use to indicate that caffeine is safe to consume in the amounts commonly found in foods and beverages. The FDA allows caffeine to be added to cola drinks.

## 4.8 Recommendation and conclusions

Caffeine is the perfect money-making drug. First, it has very desirable stimulatory effects on the central nervous system. Second, you cannot consume too much at one time because the drug produces undesirable nervous system effects. Third, you cannot stop drinking it because you will get a headache. Fourth, the half-life of the drug is relatively short, so that you must go back for more. Fifth, you don't lose your craving for it. And finally, it is a naturally occurring substance with a long history of use that is recognized by the regulatory authorities as being safe. The coffee, tea, and cola industries benefit enormously from our desire for this drug.

Each of us should be aware of our dose–response to caffeine and limit our consumption accordingly. If you are pregnant, think about whether you want your fetus swimming in caffeine and its metabolites.

## 4.9 More information and references

### 4.9.1 Slide presentation

■  A Small Dose of Caffeine presentation material. Online. Available HTTP: <http://www.crcpress.com/e_products/> and follow the links to downloads and then the catalog number TF1691.
    Web site contains presentation material related to the health effects of caffeine.

## 4.9.2 European, Asian, and international agencies

■   International Food Information Council (IFIC) Foundation. Online. Available HTTP: <http://ific.org/> (accessed: 2 April 2003).
   IFIC's mission is to communicate science-based information on food safety and nutrition to health and nutrition professionals, educators, journalists, government officials and others providing information to consumers. IFIC is supported primarily by the broad-based food, beverage, and agricultural industries.

■   England – Department of Health – Committee on toxicity of chemicals in food consumer products and the environment – Statement on the reproductive effects of caffeine. Online. Available HTTP: <http://www.doh.gov.uk/sacn/pdf/200106caffeine.pdf> (accessed: 2 April 2003).
   Excellent report on the reproductive effects of caffeine.

## 4.9.3 North American agencies

■   US MEDLINEplus Health Information. Online. Available HTTP: <http://www.nlm.nih.gov/medlineplus/caffeine.html> (accessed: 2 April 2003).
   Medline has multiple references on caffeine, including a number of useful web-based links.

■   US Food and Drug Administration (FDA) – Perplexities Of Pregnancy. Online. Available HTTP: <http://www.cfsan.fda.gov/~dms/wh-preg2.html> (accessed: 9 April 2003).
   This FDA document provided information on caffeine during pregnancy and advises "pregnant women to eliminate caffeine from their diets".

■   US Center for the Evaluation of Risks to Human Reproduction. Online. Available HTTP: <http://cerhr.niehs.nih.gov/genpub/topics/caffeine-ccae.html> (accessed: 2 April 2003).
   The US National Toxicology Program (NTP) and the National Institute of Environmental Health Sciences (NIEHS) have established the NTP Center for the Evaluation of Risks to Human Reproduction in 1998. The Center provides scientifically based, uniform assessments of the potential for adverse effects on reproduction and development caused by agents to which humans may be exposed.

## 4.9.4 Non-government organizations

■   Center for Science in the Public Interest – Nutrition Action. Online. Available HTTP: <http://www.cspinet.org/nah/caffeine.htm> (accessed: 2 April 2003).
   Article on caffeine and its health effects.

■   March of Dimes – Caffeine in Pregnancy Fact Sheet. Online. Available HTTP: <http://www.marchofdimes.com/aboutus/681_1148.asp> (accessed: 9 April 2003).
   March of Dimes has a number of fact sheets including this one on caffeine.

■   I Need Coffee: Non-commercial Caffeination Information. Online. Available HTTP: <http://www.ineedcoffee.com/> (accessed: 2 April 2003).
   A humorous but factual look at coffee consumption.

- In Pursuit of Tea. Online. Available HTTP: <http://www.inpursuitoftea.com/> (accessed: 2 April 2003).
  Company web site dedicated to "Exploring remote regions of the world to supply the finest True Teas".
- Caffeine – The Vaults of Erowid. Online. Available HTTP: <http://www.erowid.org/chemicals/caffeine/caffeine.shtml> (accessed: 2 April 2003).
  The Erowid web site has a wide range of information on caffeine.

### 4.9.5 References

- Caffeine and Pregnancy. Organization of Teratology Information Services (OTIS). Online. Available HTTP: <http://www.otispregnancy.org/pdf/caffeine.pdf> (accessed: 5 April 2003).
- *The World of Caffeine – The Science and Culture of the World's Most Popular Drug*, by:
  Bennett Alan Weinberg and Bonnie K. Bealer. Routledge, New York, 2001.
- *Caffeine & Health*, by Jack E. James. Academic Press – Harcourt Brace Jovanovish, Publishers, New York, 1991.

# Chapter 5

# Nicotine

## Contents

## 5.1 Dossier

**Name:** nicotine
**Use:** pesticide, drug in tobacco
**Source:** tobacco
**Recommended daily intake:** none (not essential)
**Absorption:** lung, skin, stomach (poor), intestine (better), (poor absorption in the stomach because nicotine is a strong base)
**Sensitive individuals:** fetus, children
**Toxicity/symptoms:** dependency producing, acute effects: nausea, vomiting, salivation, diarrhea, dizziness, mental confusion, weakness
**Regulatory facts:** RfD (none), $LD_{50}$ 10 mg/kg
**General facts:** long history of use, produces dependency in user
**Environmental:** growing demand for cigarettes in developing countries
**Recommendations:** avoid

## 5.2 Case studies

### 5.2.1 "The divine origin of tobacco"

Tobacco was a powerful medicine for the first people of the Americas. Native Californian tribes trace the origins of tobacco to sacred immortals that first inhabited the land. The immortals gave tobacco to the humans to heal and guide them from the ancient past to the present and beyond: it was part of creation. Medicine doctors and shaman relied upon tobacco for guidance, a source of strength and part of the healing ritual. Tobacco was sacred, not to be rapidly consumed in the doorway of a back alley. As Julian Lang suggested, the warning on a pack of cigarettes should be "Use of this product should be restricted to prayerful or religious activity, or social activity which reflects aspects of the Creation" (Lang, 1997).

### 5.2.2 Green tobacco sickness

Green tobacco sickness (GTS) afflicts workers harvesting tobacco when nicotine is absorbed through the skin from handling wet tobacco leaves. Workers report symptoms of nausea, vomiting, weakness, dizziness, headache, and, depending on the amount of exposure, decreases in heart rate and blood pressure. These are the classic signs of nicotine poisoning. This illness often lasts for several days, and some workers require hospital treatment. In the fields, the workers' clothes become wet from moisture on the tobacco leaves, and most workers do not use gloves or protective clothing. Workers that use tobacco products are less likely to suffer from GTS because of tolerance to the effects of nicotine. Another interesting observation is that older workers are less likely to develop GTS, possibly because younger workers sensitive to nicotine drop out of the work force. Appropriate worker education about the absorption of nicotine through the skin and use of protective clothing would reduce the incidence of GTS. For more information see Morbidity Mortality Weekly Report on GTS (reference below).

## 5.3 Introduction and history

Nicotine is a potent drug with a long history of use and enormous effects on our society. From a toxicology perspective, nicotine is a naturally occurring pesticide in tobacco, a powerful drug with multiple nervous system effects, and thus cigarettes are a drug delivery device.

Nicotine was isolated from tobacco leaves (*Nicotiana tabacum*) in 1828, but the powerful effects of nicotine were already well recognized. The tobacco plant is native to the Americas and its use as a medicine and stimulant goes back at least 2000 years and most likely many millennia before that. Fine temple carvings show Mayan priests enjoying the benefits of this drug from smoking tobacco through a pipe (Figure 5.1). Tobacco appears to part of the healing arts and sacred rituals of many of the native peoples of the Americas.

There are various theories of how tobacco was introduced to Europe, but undoubtedly Christopher Columbus and his crews sampled this native weed and

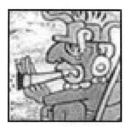

**Figure 5.1.** Mayan priest smoking tobacco, 1000 BC. Ancient temple carvings depict Mayan priests in Central America smoking tobacco through a pipe. Tobacco leaves became widespread in medicine for use on wounds as a means of reducing pain. Later the Aztecs incorporated smoke inhalation into religious rituals.

succumbed to its spell. Once introduced into Europe, tobacco use in pipes and as cigars spread rapidly. Some thought it was powerful medicine and might even cure the Plague, while others saw it as an evil and nasty habit.

> We found a man in a canoe going from Santa Maria to Fernandia. He had with him . . . some dried leaves which are in high value among them, for a quantity of it was brought to me at San Salvador.
> Christopher Columbus' Journal, 15 October 1492

The habit of tobacco use is directly related to the biological effects of nicotine. While people in the 1500s did not understand the mechanisms behind the complex physiological effects of nicotine, they certainly felt and appreciated its stimulant and relaxing properties. The desire to consume nicotine is encouraged not only by these seemingly pleasant effects, but also by the need to avoid the unpleasant effects of not having nicotine in your blood. Tobacco consumption became a powerful habit that has influenced society in countless ways.

The influence of tobacco and nicotine started early and continues today. By the early 1600s tobacco farming had become an important cash crop for export to Europe by the new colonies in North America. Some historians believe the colonies would not have prospered without this source of money. Tobacco is a demanding crop to grow, and as tobacco farming spread south there was a growing demand for workers. In the 1700s tobacco plantation farmers began importing African slaves to work the farms. Tobacco became important not only for local economies, but also for national governments as soon as it became apparent that one could tax the people's habit. It is only relatively recently that society has looked at the true cost of tobacco consumption.

It took many years to refine and develop tobacco consumption as a means of drug delivery. Tobacco consumption was initially confined to chewing or smoking with a pipe or cigar. Cigarettes were invented in 1614 by beggars in Seville, Spain, who collected scraps of cigars and rolled the tobacco into small pieces of paper. Cigarette consumption grew gradually in popularity, but they were expensive to produce until 1880 when a machine to roll cigarettes was patented. This invention ushered in much cheaper cigarettes and major tobacco corporations.

The undesirable health effects of tobacco consumption were not entirely unrecognized. By 1890, 26 states had passed laws banning the sale of cigarettes to minors. Cigarette consumption increased steadily, spurred along by both world wars and relentless marketing by the tobacco companies. In 1964, the US Surgeon General issued a report linking smoking with lung cancer and heart disease, which started a slow recognition of the true cost of smoking and began a decline in consumption. It was not until 1994 that the US Food and Drug Administration officially determined that nicotine was a dependency-producing drug. The US Supreme Court subsequently ruled that the FDA could not regulate nicotine as a drug. However, all this attention did encourage legal action that resulted in the tobacco companies paying billions of dollars to cover health care costs. While tobacco consumption is declining in North America and parts of Europe, it continues to increase in many parts of the world that have yet to recognize the costs both to the individual and ultimately to society.

The widespread personal consumption of nicotine is not its only role. In 1763 it was first used as an insecticide. The potent nervous system effects of nicotine kill or deter insects. Nicotine is extracted from tobacco leaves by steam or solvent treatment and then sprayed on vegetation where it is readily absorbed by insects.

## 5.4 Biological properties

Nicotine has a range of physiological effects and has provided researchers with many insights into nervous system function. It is readily absorbed through the skin and lungs, but because it is a strong base is not well absorbed in the acid environment of the stomach. Nicotine travels from the lungs to the brain in about 7 seconds; thus each puff produces a reinforcing effect. The positive effects of nicotine are associated with a complex balance of stimulation and relaxation. For example, depending on the dose, it can increase or decrease the heart rate. One of the most prominent reactions of first time users is nausea and vomiting. This is due to stimulation of both central and peripheral nervous systems that triggers a vomiting reaction. The underlying mechanism of action is its effect on acetylcholine-like receptors, sometimes referred to as nicotinic receptors.

Nicotine is metabolized in the liver, lung, and kidney. It has a relatively short half-life of about 2 hours, which greatly contributes to the desire to smoke in an effort to restore the blood nicotine levels. Its primary metabolite is cotinine, which has a much longer half-life than nicotine. Nicotine and its metabolites are readily excreted in the urine. Because of cotinine's longer half-life, insurance companies will typically test urine or blood samples for cotinine to determine if someone is smoking. Nicotine is also excreted in the breast milk of nursing mothers, with heavy smokers having up to 0.5 mg per liter of milk. Given the infant's small size, this can represent a significant dose of nicotine.

The skin absorption of nicotine and subsequent adverse effects make it an effective pesticide. Nicotine poisoning occurs primarily by children coming into contact with nicotine insecticides or tobacco products.

## 5.5 Health effects

Smoking is a custom loathsome to the eye, hateful to the nose, harmful to the brain, dangerous to the lungs, and in the black, stinking fume thereof nearest resembling the horrible Stygian smoke of the pit that is bottomless.
James I of England, A Counterblaste to Tobacco, 1604.

Nicotine is a highly toxic drug, with only 60 mg being lethal to an adult. The average cigarette contains 8 to 9 mg of nicotine; so one pack of cigarettes contains enough nicotine to kill your average adult, to say nothing of a child. Depending on technique, a smoker receives about 1 mg of nicotine per cigarette. The effects of nicotine are complex but are similar to acetylcholine poisoning. Acute effects of nicotine poisoning include nausea, vomiting, salivation, diarrhea, dizziness, mental confusion, and weakness. At high levels of exposure, nicotine causes decreased blood pressure, difficulty breathing, irregular pulse, convulsions, respiratory failure, and death.

Nicotine is probably the most addictive drug readily available to the average person. The nicotinic effects from smoking are highly reinforcing, with some users comparing the effects to cocaine or amphetamine. Regular smokers consume nicotine for stimulation but also to avoid the withdrawal effects. The withdrawal effects are well known and include irritability, anxiety, restlessness, impatience, increased appetite, and weight gain. Nicotine patches are used to maintain a steady-state blood level of nicotine and thus reduce the desire to smoke. Nicotine gum and now nicotine drinks are produced as an alternative to smoking.

Nicotine also affects the developing fetus. Adverse effects of chronic nicotine consumption during pregnancy include reduced infant birth weight, attention deficit disorders, and other cognitive problems. Nicotine receptors are expressed early during development, and it is not clear what other effects nicotine exposure during development has on the fetus.

The health effects of nicotine cannot be entirely separated from the effects of cigarettes as a whole. Nicotine keeps people smoking, but the many other compounds that are inhaled when smoking typically result in respiratory disease, cardiovascular disease, and lung cancer.

## 5.6 Reducing exposure

> To cease smoking is the easiest thing I ever did. I ought to know, I've done it a thousand times.
>
> Mark Twain

Given the serious health effects from cigarette smoking, primarily maintained by the addictive properties of nicotine, the best advice is not to start. Despite the obvious health problems and cost to society, large numbers of young people start smoking each year.

All nicotine-containing products should be handled with care and kept out of the reach of children.

## 5.7 Regulatory standards

The US FDA tried but failed to win approval to regulate nicotine, and the US Congress has not stepped forward to allow the FDA to regulate this very potent drug.

## 5.8 Recommendation and conclusions

Nicotine is a very potent drug, highly addictive when regularly consumed, and its use should be avoided.

## 5.9 More information and references

### 5.9.1 Slide presentation

- A Small Dose of Nicotine presentation material. Online. Available HTTP: <http://www.crcpress.com/e_products/> and follow the links to downloads and then the catalog number TF1691.
  Web site contains presentation material related to the health effects of nicotine.

### 5.9.2 European, Asian, and international agencies

- England – Department of Health – Scientific Committee on Tobacco and Health (SCOTH). Online. Available HTTP: < http://www.doh.gov.uk/scoth/> (accessed: 2 April 2003).
  "SCOTH advises the UK Chief Medical Officer on the health effects of smoking."
- Society for Research on Nicotine and Tobacco. Online. Available HTTP: <http://www.srnt.org/> (accessed: 2 April 2003).
  "An international Society with a mission to stimulate the generation of new knowledge concerning nicotine in all its manifestations – from molecular to societal."
- World Health Organization (WHO). Online. Available HTTP: <http://www.who.int/health_topics/tobacco/en/> (accessed: 2 April 2003).
  Covers tobacco and international efforts to track and reduce use of tobacco.
- National Tobacco Information Online System (NATIONS). Online. Available HTTP: <http://apps.nccd.cdc.gov/nations/about/NATIONS.asp> (accessed: 2 April 2003).
  "The National Tobacco Information Online System (NATIONS) is an electronically integrated information system containing country-specific information on a wide variety of tobacco control issues."

### 5.9.3 North American agencies

- Health Canada – Tobacco (CDC). Online. Available HTTP: <http://www.hc-sc.gc.ca/hecs-sesc/tobacco/index.html> (accessed: 9 April 2003).
  Health Canada information on the health effects of tobacco.
- US Centers for Disease Control and Prevention (CDC). Online. Available HTTP: <http://www.cdc.gov/health/tobacco.htm> (accessed: 2 April 2003).
  Site has multiple listing on health, tobacco, and nicotine.
- US National Institute on Drug Abuse (NIDA). Online. Available HTTP: <http://www.drugabuse.gov/drugpages/nicotine.html> (accessed: 2 April 2003).
  Site has general information on nicotine.

### 5.9.4 Non-government organizations

- Society for Neuroscience (SfN). Online. Available HTTP: <http://www.sfn.org/content/Publications/BrainBriefings/nicotine.html> (accessed: 2 April 2003).

This article is part of the SfN series on Brain Briefing, this one covers nicotine and the brain.

■ Tobacco and Nicotine – The Vaults of Erowid. Online. Available HTTP: <http://www.erowid.org/plants/tobacco/tobacco.shtml> (accessed: 2 April 2003). Site has a wide range of information on tobacco and nicotine.

### 5.9.5 References

■ Lang, J. (1997). The devine origin of tobacco. Winds of Change, 12(3), 55–59.
■ MMWR (1993). Green tobacco sickness in tobacco harvesters – Kentucky, 1992. Vol. 42, (13), 237. Online. Available HTTP: <http://www.cdc.gov/mmwr/preview/mmwrhtml/00020119.htm> (accessed: 5 July 2003).

# Chapter 6

# Pesticides

## Contents

- Dossier – insecticides
- Dossier – herbicides
- Case studies
- Introduction and history
- Biological properties
- Health effects
- Reducing exposure
- Regulatory standards
- Recommendation and conclusions
- More information and references

## 6.1 Dossier – insecticides

**Use:** kill insects
**Source:** synthetic chemistry, plants
**Recommended daily intake:** none (not essential)
**Absorption:** intestine, inhalation, skin
**Sensitive individuals:** fetus, children, and elderly
**Toxicity/symptoms:** nervous system, range of problems depending on chemical
**Regulatory facts:** RfDs exist for many insecticides. Regulated by EPA.
**General facts:** billions of pounds used every year in agriculture and around the home
**Environmental:** pesticides are used globally; some are very persistent in the environment

## 6.2 Dossier – herbicides

**Use:** kill or injure plants
**Source:** synthetic chemistry
**Recommended daily intake:** none (not essential)
**Absorption:** intestine, inhalation, skin
**Sensitive individuals:** fetus, children
**Toxicity/symptoms:** varies
**Regulatory facts:** RfDs exist for many insecticides. Regulated by EPA.
**General facts:** long history of use, now being used in combination with genetically modified plants
**Environmental:** global environmental
**Recommendations:** avoid, consider alternatives, integrated pest management

## 6.3 Case studies

### 6.3.1 Cats, dogs, and fleas

Fleas are very small and annoying blood-sucking pests, capable of spreading serious human diseases. We come in contact with fleas primarily through our pet cats and dogs. Fleas have a complex life cycle and reproduce rapidly, so flea control is an important issue in any household with pets. A common insecticide used to kill fleas on cats is imidacloprid. This insecticide is also used to control sucking insects such as aphids, whiteflies, termites and a range of other soil insects, and some beetles. It is also very toxic to bees. Imidacloprid is toxic to the nervous system, causing an overstimulation of acetylcholine nicotinic nerves, resulting in the insect's paralysis and death. When used to control fleas, it is typically applied to the back of the cat's neck. Imidacloprid is absorbed through the skin and circulates in the blood. The flea dies after biting the cat and consuming the cat's blood, which contains this toxic chemical. The cat appears to be unaffected by this chemical primarily because it receives a very small amount of pesticide relative to the cat's body weight. Effects of overexposure on the cat would include muscle weakness, fatigue, and twitching. The flea, because of its very small size, receives a much larger dose because of its small body weight. The average flea weighs between 0.5 mg and 1 mg and can double its body weight when feeding. It takes only a very small amount of pesticide in the blood of the animal to kill the flea.

### 6.3.2 Farm worker illness from pesticides

Agricultural pesticide use in the United States is about 1.2 billion pounds of active ingredient each year and total pesticide use is close to 6 billion pounds. Worldwide agricultural pesticide use is about 5 billion pounds of active ingredient each year. The active pesticide chemical is often less that 1% of the material applied; these estimates do not include chemicals used to dissolve or carry the active pesticide chemical. Determining the amount used is difficult because there is no national requirement to report pesticide use. Commercial agriculture uses approximately 60%

of pesticides and the rest is used by homeowners, government, and industry on lawns and gardens and inside buildings.

The use of pesticides in large agricultural applications requires training and knowledge to ensure that worker exposure is minimized. Carbofuran (N-methyl carbamate) is a broad-spectrum insecticide used on rice, alfalfa, table and wine grapes, and cotton. Carbamate insecticides inhibit cholinesterase, which causes an increase in acetylcholine. Elevated acetylcholine levels cause tremor, paralysis, and death of the insect. Farm workers come into contact with pesticides during the application or from entering the fields after application. When carbofuran is used on cotton, there is a 48-hour waiting period before farm workers are allowed to enter the field. This is to allow the carbamate to dissipate and degrade to ensure that worker exposure to the active pesticide is minimized. In 1998, an airplane applied carbofuran to a cotton field in the state of California. Within hours of the spraying of carbofuran, 34 farm workers entered the cotton field to continue weeding. Several hours later the workers became ill with symptoms, including nausea, headache, eye irritation, muscle weakness, salivation, and decreased heart rate as well as other complaints. The symptoms are consistent with poisoning from a cholinesterase inhibitor. The majority of the workers were hospitalized and decontaminated, including decontamination of their clothing. Several of the workers went home without decontaminating, which raises the issue of family exposure to pesticide on the clothing. Infants or young children are most susceptible and vulnerable to take-home exposures from the workplace. More information is available on this incident from the US Centers for Disease Control report (MMWR, 1998).

## 6.4 Introduction and history

> Chlordane – America's leading lawn and garden insecticide. Used extensively by pest control operators for termite control, because of its long lasting effectiveness.
>
> Velsicol Chemical Corporation, Advertisement, 1959.
>
> The US EPA lists chlordane as a persistent bioaccumulative toxic chemical. In 1978, the EPA cancelled use of chlordane on food crops and by 1988 all use was banned.

The function of a pesticide is to destroy some form of life. Many plants and animals have developed sophisticated pesticides to protect themselves from other plants and animals bent on doing them harm. Humans used these naturally occurring pesticides as a starting point and, in the twentieth century, through chemical synthesis, developed a remarkable array of deadly pesticides designed to kill bacteria, fungi, plants, animals, and even other humans. This chapter will only skim the surface of pesticides, for it is a large and complex subject that ranges from chemistry, biological mechanisms of action, environmental concerns, government regulation, business, and indeed our very civilization.

The two largest classes of pesticides are insecticides, designed to kill insects, and herbicides, designed to kill plants. Other major pesticide groups include fungicides, rodenticides, and antimicrobials. Although many medications are in effect pesticides, because they kill invading organisms, such as parasitic worms, bacteria, and viruses, pharmaceuticals are not defined as pesticides and are regulated separately. Antibiotics are pesticides directed at bacteria. They are generally safe for humans and animals to consume at dosages prescribed by trained physicians. However, as with many pesticides, antibiotics can cause problems. They are generally not specific to only one kind of bacteria and thus kill helpful bacteria. Even more serious, bacteria adapt to the antibiotic and become resistant to its effects.

One of the first pesticides was sulfur, used by the Chinese in 1000 BC to control bacteria and mold (fungus). Sulfur is still widely used today in the wine industry to control unwanted growth in wine barrels and is commonly added to wine to kill unwanted yeast. The Chinese also pioneered the use of arsenic-containing compounds to control insects. Arsenic has a long history of use both as an insecticide and herbicide, and then as medicine (see chapter on arsenic). Arsenic trioxide was used as a weed killer in the late 1800s and lead arsenate was a very important insecticide particularly in orchards in the early 1900s. Some of the first concerns about pesticide safety were raised over lead arsenate residue on fruit, and to this day some orchard soils remain contaminated with lead and arsenic. In the late 1600s nicotine was recognized as a potent insecticide and an extract from tobacco leaves was sprayed on plants. Even today certain arsenic compounds are used as herbicides and as wood preservatives.

Plants have provided several other important pesticides. The group of insecticides called pyrethrums was harvested and refined from chrysanthemums. The plant nux vomica contains strychnine, which was used to kill rodents. Rotenone, another important insecticide was extracted from the root of *Derris eliptica*. Plant extracts were useful, but difficult to purify and obtain in quantity. Significant increases in the use of pesticides occurred with advances in synthetic chemistry and our understanding of biology.

Synthetic chemistry advanced rapidly in the 1930s and by the early 1940s a range of new pesticides had been developed, including organochlorines like DDT (Figure 6.1). In 1937 the first organophosphorus compounds were synthesized by a group of German chemists. These very potent compounds were kept secret during the Second World War and developed as potential chemical warfare agents. Unfortunately, these compounds were subsequently developed and used as warfare agents and even utilized by terrorists. After the war, this class of compounds became an important group of insecticides following extensive and continuing research and development. Along with a desire to develop new insecticides was an equally strong effort to develop new herbicides to increase food production and as potential warfare agents. In 1946, the first commercially available chlorine-based herbicides were marketed to kill broad-leaved plants. This class of compounds includes 2,4-D, 2,4,5-T, and its well-known contaminant TCDD (dioxin). These herbicides were extensively utilized in agriculture, to clear roadsides and right of ways, and in warfare to clear enemy hiding sites. Dioxin contamination ultimately led to the ban of 2,4,5-T by the US EPA, but 2,4-D is still one of the most widely used herbicides.

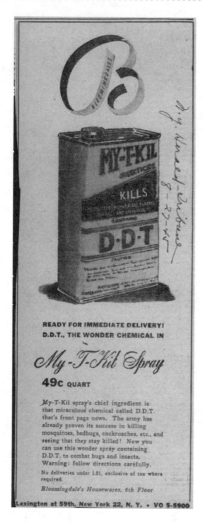

**Figure 6.1.** DDT advertisement in the *New York Herald Tribune*, 1945. With permission from Medicine and Madison Avenue. 2002. Rare Book, Manuscript, and Special Collections Library, Duke University. (http://scriptorium.lib.duke.edu/mma/)

We learned through bitter experience the necessity of regulating the manufacture and use of pesticides. Regulation was initially focused on protecting the consumer from pesticide residue on food, but it was also apparent that protection was needed for the workers applying or working near pesticides. Congress passed the first federal act specifically dealing with pesticides in 1947. This act, the Federal Insecticide, Fungicide, and Rodenticide Act (FIFRA), was the first attempt at requiring that pesticides be both safe and effective. Rachel Carson's *Silent Spring*, published in 1962, marks a turning point in our appreciation of the effects of chemicals on human and environmental health. In 1972 the US Environmental Protection Agency was formed and given authority for the registration of pesticides based on evaluating and weighing estimated risks and benefits. In 1996 the Food Quality Protection Act passed by Congress required that special consideration be given to children's exposure and special sensitivity to pesticides and other

**Table 6.1 Pesticide use in the United States**

| Type | Billions of pounds | % |
|------|--------------------|-----|
| Conventional pesticides (agriculture) | 0.97 | 21 |
| Other pesticide chemicals (sulfur . . . ) | 0.26 | 6 |
| Wood preservatives | 0.66 | 14 |
| Specialty biocides | 0.27 | 6 |
| Chlorine/hypochlorites | 2.46 | 53 |
| Total | 4.63 | 100 |

Chlorine and hypochlorites are used in water purification.

chemicals. This act requires extra safety factors for children unless it can be shown that they are not needed for a particular chemical.

Both the volume of use and the amount of money spent demonstrates our dependency on pesticides. In 1997, the EPA reported that 4.6 billion pounds of pesticide were used in the United States, which is equivalent to 4.4 pounds per person. Of this, almost 1 billion pounds, with 600 different active ingredients, were used in agriculture and another 0.26 billion pounds used by homeowners, government, and industry on lawns and gardens. This use alone amounts to an expenditure of $11.9 billion, of which $8.3 billion is spent by agriculture. Wood preservatives add another 0.66 billion pounds and disinfectants 2.5 billion pounds (Table 6.1). Worldwide 5.7 billion pounds of agricultural-based pesticides were used at a cost of $37 billion (see presentation for details).

The history, use, development, toxicology, and regulation of pesticides make a fascinating story on many different levels. From a toxicology perspective, pesticides function because of dose–response, and it is the sensitivity of the individual, particularly children, to the more subtle effects of pesticide exposure that is now driving the need to regulate pesticides more tightly and to reduce exposure. People worldwide are recognizing the impact of pesticides on the environment. We probably need some pesticides to feed the world population; the challenge is to use these agents that are designed to kill, prudently, and with knowledge of their benefits and potential harm. Past experience teaches us that we need to reduce unnecessary pesticide use, find safer and more selective pest management tools, and protect sensitive populations from exposure.

## 6.5 Biological properties

### 6.5.1 Introduction

Pesticide exposure can occur through foods, drinking water, home use of pesticides in the garden, from indoor insect control, or through occupational exposure, particularly in an agricultural setting. Pesticides illustrate the basic principles of toxicology: dose–response and individual sensitivity. Designed to kill – and for insecticides this usually means toxicity to the nervous system – a small amount of pesticide is fatal to an insect primarily because of the insect's small size and high

**Table 6.2 Comparison of body weight and dose**

|  | Body weight | Amount of chemical needed for a dose of 10 mg/kg |
|---|---|---|
| Adult | 70 kg (150 lbs) | 700 mg |
| Child | 10 kg (22 lbs) | 100 mg |
| Insect | 1 mg | 0.00001 mg (1/100 000 mg) |

rate of metabolism. For an insect a small exposure can represent a very large dose on a body weight basis. This same small amount is relatively less harmful to an animal of much larger size, because it is a small dose based on body weight. However, it is this same principle that makes children more vulnerable than adults. Table 6.2 illustrates how much of a chemical is needed to achieve the same dose for an adult, a child, and an insect. Size is a very important factor. While a single exposure can be deadly, repetitive exposures to pesticides can also cause adverse effects as well.

There is no perfect pesticide. Pesticides work by interfering with some basic biological function essential for life, and because living organisms share many common biological mechanisms, pesticides are never specific to just one species of life. While killing a true pest, pesticides also kill other organisms that are either desirable or at least not undesirable, and we have a far from perfect understanding of what is undesirable. The ideal pesticide would be highly specific, quick acting, and degrade rapidly to non-toxic materials in the environment.

### 6.5.2 Insecticides

Most modern chemical insecticides act by poisoning the nervous system. The central and peripheral nervous system of insects is fundamentally similar to that of mammals. This means that given sufficient exposure insecticides will adversely affect human health. Insecticides are lethal to insects because of the high dose (exposure relative to body size). The similarities of nervous system structure make it impossible to design highly specific insecticides using this mode of action, and so there are always a number of non-target organisms that will be affected. New generations of insecticides are designed to be as specific as possible with the least amount of environmental persistence. We will examine the most prominent classes of insecticides – organochlorines, pyrethroids, organophosphates, and carbamates – in more detail.

Organochlorines, which include DDT, illustrate many of the wrongs about insecticides while having the advantage of being cheap to manufacture and effective against serious target species. They are largely banned in North America and Europe, but are still an important class of insecticides in developing countries. DDT, for example, is still being manufactured for export in the United States. The chemical structure of organochlorines is diverse but they all contain chlorine, which places them in a larger class of compounds called chlorinated hydrocarbons. At one time organochlorines were thought to be ideal because they are very stable, persistent and slow to degrade in the environment, lipid soluble (therefore readily taken up by insects), and apparently harmless to mammals. It eventually became clear that persistence and fat solubility were actually very undesirable and that the compounds could have long-term health effects on mammals. These highly persistent and lipid-soluble chemicals are passed up the food chain where they bioaccumulate in fat and are passed on to nursing infants of both humans and other animals. The global transport of these chemicals results in the contamination of wildlife around the globe including in Arctic and Antarctic regions. A decline in the number of predatory birds was one of the first signs of the unintended consequences of DDT. These birds accumulated DDT from eating other mammals that had been exposed to DDT. Unexpectedly, DDT caused a thinning of the birds' eggshells and the death of their developing young. From the perspective of the nervous system, organochlorines disrupt the movement of ions such as $Ca^{++}$, $Cl^-$, $Na^+$ and $K^+$ into and out of the nerve cells, which leads to hypersensitivity and ultimately death. Depending on the structure of the chemical, it may also have other effects on the nervous system. Organochlorine insecticides provide many important lessons about the desirable and undesirable properties of pesticides.

Organophosphates and carbamates have very different chemical structures but share a similar mechanism of action and will be examined here as one class of insecticides. Organophosphates were initially developed in the 1940s as highly toxic biological warfare agents (nerve gases). Modern derivatives, including sarin, soman, and VX were stockpiled by the military of various countries and continue to present some difficult disposal problems. Researchers created many different organophosphates in their search for ones that would target selected species and are less toxic to mammals. When the organophosphate parathion was first used as a replacement for DDT, there were a number of human deaths because workers failed to appreciate the parathion's toxicity after working with much less acutely toxic DDT. Adequate worker protection and training is essential when working with organophosphates. The problem with organophosphates and carbamates is that they affect an important neurotransmitter common to both insects and mammals. This neurotransmitter, acetylcholine, is extensively used to communicate between nerve cells. After the acetylcholine is released from one cell to initiate communication with another cell it must be removed to stop the communication. This class of insecticides blocks an enzyme specifically designed to break down the no-longer-needed acetylcholine. The enzyme that breaks down acetylcholine is called acetylcholinesterase, and this class of insecticides is commonly referred to as anti-acetylcholinesterase to acknowledge that they block this enzyme. Structural differences between the various organophosphates and carbamates affect the efficiency and degree to which the acetylcholinesterase is blocked. For example, the very potent nerve gases are highly efficient and permanently block acetylcholinesterase, while the more commonly used pesticides only block acetylcholinesterase temporarily. The human toxicity of these pesticides presents significant human health hazards, and researchers have continued to develop new insecticides.

The newest class of insecticide, pyrethroids, is loosely based upon the naturally occurring pyrethrum derived from chrysanthemum flowers. Synthetic pyrethroids were developed in the 1980s but the naturally occurring pyrethrum was first commercially used in the 1800s. The chemical structure of pyrethroids is quite different from organochlorines and organophosphates, but the primary site of action remains the nervous system. Pyrethroids affect the movement of $Na^+$ (sodium ions) into and out of nerve cells, causing the nerve cells to become hypersensitive. Structure differences in pyrethroids can influence their toxicity toward specific insects and to mammals. The use of synthetic pyrethroids has increased significantly over the last 20 years. Synthetic pyrethroids are more persistent in the environment than natural pyrethrum, which is unstable to light and breaks down very quickly.

### 6.5.3 Herbicides

Herbicides, used to kill or damage a plant, are the most rapidly growing segment of pesticides. Prior to the 1930s, herbicides were non-specific and often very toxic to humans as well as other animals. In the 1930s, in parallel with the development of new insecticides, researchers discovered several chemicals that selectively killed plants. These chemicals are now widely used to increase food production and have been used in warfare. Herbicides come in a variety of chemical structures and mechanisms of action, so they will be discussed in only general terms. Interested readers are referred to the many web sites and extensive literature on herbicides (see below and the presentation).

The most famous (or infamous) of herbicides are the chlorophenoxy compounds that include 2,4-D, 2,4,5-T, and its contaminant TCDD. This herbicide mixture, sometimes called Agent Orange, was widely used to kill broad-leaved plants in agriculture fields, along roadsides, and right of ways for power lines. It was also extensively used as a chemical warfare agent to kill unwanted vegetation. The mechanism of action of this class of chemicals is poorly understood but they appear to interact with plant growth hormones. Improvements in the manufacturing process of chlorophenoxy compounds and the cancellation of 2,4,5-T registration has reduced contaminants such as TCDD.

Paraquat and the related chemical diquat are nonselective herbicides that are also toxic to mammals. Occupational or accidental exposure to paraquat can be from oral ingestion, dermal exposure, or inhalation, all of which can cause serious illness or death. While seldom used in the United States, paraquat is still widely used in developing countries. At one time it was used to kill marijuana plants, but a number of fatalities were observed when marijuana contaminated with paraquat was inhaled.

There are many other herbicides in widespread use with a range of actions including alachlor, glyphosate, and atrazine. Herbicides are now an essential part of the agriculture business and thought by some to be necessary to feed the world's growing population. A serious limitation of many herbicides is a lack of specificity; in other words the herbicide damages the crop of interest. To solve this problem, the manufacturers of herbicides have used biotechnology techniques to make herbicide-resistant crops. For example, the Monsanto company produced the glyphosate-based herbicide called RoundUp. The company then manufactured a genetically modified soybean resistant to the herbicide. The genetically modified soybean, called RoundUp Ready, is now widely planted, which has the effect of increasing the sale of Monsanto herbicide. Genetically engineered plants raise many new health and safety questions.

## 6.5.4 Fungicides, rodenticides, and molluscicides

Fungicides were developed to control the fungi and mold that in various forms are all around us and even on us. Initially, fungicides consisted of sulfur, copper sulfate, mercury-based compounds and other metal-containing compounds. Chemical fungicides are now available for both medical treatment of human fungal disease and agricultural applications. Control of plant fungus is important not only because they can damage the plant but also because some fungi produce toxic chemicals (mycotoxins). One of the more interesting fungi, *Aspergillus flavus*, can contaminate nuts (e.g. peanuts) and grains (e.g. corn). This fungus produces aflatoxin, which can cause liver disease and in some situations liver cancer. Another grain fungus produces an ergot alkaloid, which can cause hallucinations. The fungicide hexachlorobenzene was widely used in the 1940s and 1950s to protect seed grain. Mercurial compounds were also used to protect seed grain from soil fungus. Both of these chemicals caused tragic human suffering when the treated seed was consumed instead of being planted. Fungicides can often be avoided through procedures to limit contamination or modify environmental conditions.

Rodenticides are a broad class of chemicals designed to kill mammals, particularly rats and mice. Compounds that inhibit blood clotting, anticoagulants, are commonly used to control rat populations. One of the first was warfarin, which is related to the plant-derived coumadin (from spoiled sweet clover). In the 1950s rats developed resistance to warfarin, which prompted the development of more potent anticoagulants. Other rodenticides include fluoroacetic acid and zinc phosphide (very toxic) and thiourea-based compounds. The primary alternative to using rodenticides is trapping.

Molluscicides are used to control slugs and snails. As molluscs, they are closely related to shellfish. The most commonly used active ingredient is metaldehyde, which disrupts the gastric organs, causing death. The material is often manufactured in the form of brightly colored pellets, which are attractive and toxic to children. The pellets are also attractive to wildlife and dogs and cats. Some manufacturers have added a bitter agent to make the products unpalatable to animals. Alternatives include trapping or catching the slugs and designing a garden that is less attractive to them, or using barriers to keep them out. Slug baits based on iron phosphate are also available and appear to be somewhat less toxic.

# 6.6 Health effects

## 6.6.1 Introduction

Three of the most important health-related issues of pesticides are (1) worker safety, (2) effects on children, and (3) unintended effects on other species and the environment. The root of these issues is that all species have certain fundamental biological similarities and no matter how hard we try, pesticides cannot be designed for just one target species. Pesticides are designed to kill, and because they are non-specific often kill or harm unintended organisms, including humans. The World Health Organization estimates that there are 3 million cases of pesticide poisoning each year with up to 220,000 deaths, largely in developing countries. In addition, the application of the pesticide is often not precise and unintended exposure occurs to organisms in the general area. Children, and indeed any young developing organisms, are particularly vulnerable to the harmful effects of a pesticide. The consequence of even low levels of exposure during development is not well understood.

Pesticide exposure can result in a range of neurological effects such as memory loss, loss of coordination, reduced speed of response, reduced visual ability, altered or uncontrollable mood and general behavior, and reduced motor skills. These symptoms are often very subtle and below what are generally recognized as a medically clinical effect. In addition, pesticide exposure can result in asthma, allergies, and hypersensitivity. Chronic exposure to pesticides can result in additional neurological effects as well as the possibility of an increased risk of cancer. In addition, the inert ingredients in many pesticide formulations include solvents that are toxic by inhalation and by skin absorption. Inert ingredients are not tested as thoroughly as active ingredients and are seldom disclosed on product labels. Thus, workers who apply pesticides and those who may be exposed do not know what chemicals they are exposed to.

The Natural Resources Defense Council (NRDC) report "Intolerable Risk: Pesticides in Our Children's Food" focused on the increased risk of the adverse effects of pesticides on children. This was in part because of the smaller size of the child relative to the adult and because of different food consumption practices. Relative to their size, children eat, drink, and breathe more than adults in part because they are growing. The use and regulation of pesticides illustrate the complexities of risk analysis and risk management and the difficulties in determining an acceptable level of exposure with acceptable risks. In the United States approximately 1 billion pounds of pesticides (with about 600 different active ingredients) are used annually in the agricultural sector, and worldwide approximately 4 billion pounds are used. There are a range of human health and environmental health effects associated with the use of pesticides.

### 6.6.2 Insecticides

As all the major insecticides affect the nervous system, the consequences of human exposure can appear similar. It is also important to distinguish between a high-dose acute poisoning and more chronic exposure at lower levels. Route of exposure is a factor in determining absorption and ultimately any health effects. The environmental effects, however, can be very different in large part due to persistence of the chemical in the environment.

Acute ingestion of organochlorines results in a loss of sensation around the mouth, hypersensitivity to light, sound and touch, dizziness, tremor, nausea, vomiting, apprehension, and confusion. Chronic exposure can cause weight loss, muscle weakness, headache, anxiety, and a range of other neurological complaints. For humans, DDT was thought to be relatively safe because it was poorly absorbed through the skin. It is not uncommon to see pictures of people being dusted with DDT to kill insects and demonstrate its safety. Oral ingestion of approximately 10 mg/kg would produce acute signs of poisoning. However, acute effects of organochlorines were not the problem. DDT was banned, along with most of the organochlorines, because of their environmental persistence and accumulation in the fat of animals, including humans. Another organochlorine worthy of individual mention is Kepone or chlordecone. In 1975, over 70 workers manufacturing Kepone in Hopewell, Virginia, developed a variety of neurological effects, most prominent of which became know as the "Kepone shakes". Symptoms usually started about 30 days after first exposure to Kepone. Subsequent testing also revealed a decrease in sperm count and reduced sperm motility. Ultimately, the organochlorines were found to be too environmentally toxic and organophosphates appeared to be an alternative.

Organophosphates, while environmentally more suitable than the organochlorines, present their own challenges. Foremost was their toxicity to mammals, including humans. Unlike DDT, organophosphates are absorbed through the skin, resulting in worker exposure. Acute organophosphate exposure causes signs and symptoms of excess acetylcholine, such as increased salivation and perspiration, narrowing of the pupils, nausea, diarrhea, decrease in blood pressure, muscle weakness, fatigue, and other related symptoms. Usually (if the exposure is not too great) the symptoms of acute exposure decline within days as acetylcholine levels return to normal. Some organophosphates are also responsible for a delayed neurological reaction characterized by muscle weakness in the legs and arms. Over 20,000 people were affected by this syndrome during prohibition, sometimes called "ginger jake paralysis", from drinking an alcoholic Jamaican ginger that was contaminated with a chemical called triorthocresyl phosphate (TOCP). In some patients damage was permanent. Subsequent research found that these effects could be reproduced in animals, and testing for delayed effects became required for registration of organophosphates. The human toxicity of organophosphates resulted in a steady decline in their use as alternatives were developed.

The most promising alternatives were synthetic pyrethroids. The pyrethroids, developed as derivatives of naturally occurring pyrethrum, cause hyperexcitation, aggressiveness, incoordination, whole-body tremor, and seizures. Acute exposure in humans, usually resulting from skin exposure due to poor handling procedures, usually resolves within 24 hours. While not particularly toxic to mammals, they can cause an allergic skin response in humans. Some pyrethroids may cause cancer, reproductive or developmental effects, or endocrine system effects.

### 6.6.3 Herbicides

Herbicides are designed to kill plants, not animals, and in general have lower mammalian toxicity than insecticides. Most herbicides interfere with plant hormones or enzymes that do not have any direct counterpart in animals. The most serious human health concerns have been related to contaminants of the primary chemical herbicide. There is an enormous amount of animal and some human toxicity data on 2,4-D and 2,4,5-T, but it now appears that much of this toxicity is caused by the contaminant TCDD. Military personnel exposed to Agent Orange, often contaminated with TCDD, reported birth defects, cancers, liver disease, and other illness. These concerns led to improvement in the manufacturing process to reduce TCDD contamination and ultimately to a reduction in use of 2,4-D herbicides. There is also concern that some herbicides may affect wildlife. For example, atrazine, a persistent herbicide, may adversely affect frogs. Persistence of herbicides may also contaminate surface and ground water. There is an ongoing need for more altern-atives to the use of pesticides.

### 6.6.4 Other

Fungicides have caused a number of human health disasters. In the late 1950s, approx-imately 4000 people in Turkey were poisoned by hexachlorobenzene that had been applied to seed grain to protect against soil fungus. Adults and particularly chil-dren developed diseases of the skin and bone. In Iraq, a similar incident occurred when people consumed grain coated with a mercury compound.

Rodenticides are clearly designed to kill animals and, thus, with the exception of thiourea compounds, are toxic to humans and should be avoided. Environmen-tal concerns occur when other animals consume a poisoned rodent and are in turn poisoned. Eagles, wolves, and other animals high in the food chain are particularly vulnerable.

## 6.7 Reducing exposure

With estimates of 3 million people being overtly affected by pesticides each year, there is clearly much work to be done to reduce exposures. Developing countries continue to use pesticides that have been banned in the United States and Europe.

Individually and collectively we need to examine our use of all forms of pestic-ides and consider alternatives to pesticides. Home use of pesticides is widespread, and there are also many examples of home poisoning with pesticides. Consumers who use pesticides apply them at much greater rates per acre than do farmers and other professionals. Children are at increased risk from contamination with pestic-ides from outdoors and from pesticides used inside the home. Storage and disposal of pesticides also deserves special attention. Pesticide use around the home should be avoided as much as possible by using non-chemical methods of pest control. Integrated pest management (IPM) is an approach that can significantly reduce pesticide use through prevention, monitoring, and less-toxic controls. Widely used in agriculture, landscape maintenance, and structural pest control, IPM can also be practiced by individuals in and around their homes. An IPM approach stresses proper food waste management, landscape design, plant selection, natural pest con-trols, and physical controls such as traps, barriers, and mechanical removal.

## 6.8 Regulatory standards

Experience has clearly demonstrated the need to regulate pesticide use. In the United States, the Federal Insecticide, Fungicide, and Rodenticide Act (FIFRA) was passed in 1947 and allowed the US Department of Agriculture to regulate appro-priate labeling of pesticides. The US Food and Drug Administration was given responsibility to ensure that the food supply was safe from the harmful effects of pesticides. In 1972, the administration of FIFRA was transferred to the US EPA and along with subsequent revisions greatly expanded the testing requirements before pesticides could be registered for use. Current requirements include acute toxicity testing of full formulations (with inert ingredients), but chronic and sub-chronic testing only for active ingredients. Results of these tests, which are conducted by the manufacturers and submitted to the EPA, are used to estimate potential risks to human health and the environment. There is also an international effort to harmonize regulatory standards between the United States, Europe, and Japan.

## 6.9 Recommendation and conclusions

Pesticides are widely used to ensure an adequate food supply as well as to protect our health and safety. Given the known and potential risks of pesticides, more research needs to be done to find and test alternatives to pesticides, as well as to develop pesticides that are better targeted at a particular species, be it plant, animal or fungus, and cause the least amount of environmental damage. Businesses, schools, institutions, and the home gardener that use pesticides can institute integrated pest management (IPM) policies to reduce pesticide use. An ongoing problem is the lack of data on the use of pesticides in agriculture, business, or the home. States and nations should adopt pesticide use registries to assist in the study of pesticide use patterns, pesticide-related health effects, and environmental quality studies.

## 6.10 More information and references

### 6.10.1 Slide presentation

■ A Small Dose of Pesticides presentation material. Online. Available HTTP: <http://www.crcpress.com/e_products/> and follow the links to downloads and then the catalog number TF1691.
Web site contains presentation material related to the health effects of pesticides.

### 6.10.2 European, Asian, and international agencies

■ European Union – Chemical and Pesticide Information. Online. Available HTTP: <http://europa.eu.int/comm/environment/chemicals/index.htm> (accessed: 4 April 2003).
Site contains policy and other information on the use of pesticides in agriculture.
■ World Health Organization – WHO Pesticide Evaluation Scheme (WHOPES). Online. Available HTTP: <http://www.who.int/ctd/whopes/> (accessed: 4 April 2003).
WHOPES is an "international programme which promotes and coordinates the testing and evaluation of new pesticides proposed for public health use".
■ International Programme on Chemical Safety (IPCS). Online. Available HTTP: <http://www.who.int/pcs/index.htm> (accessed: 4 April 2003).
"IPSC main roles are to establish the scientific basis for safe use of chemicals, and to strengthen national capabilities and capacities for chemical safety."

### 6.10.3 North American agencies

■ Health Canada – Pesticide Information. Online. Available HTTP: <http://www.hc-sc.gc.ca/english/search/a-z/p.html#13> (accessed: 9 April 2003).

Health Canada provided a range of information on pesticides in English and French.

■ US Environmental Protection Agency (EPA) – Office of Pesticides Programs (OPP). Online. Available HTTP: <http://www.epa.gov/pesticides/> (accessed: 4 April 2003).
OPP's mission is "to protect public health and the environment from the risks posed by pesticides and to promote safer means of pest control".

■ US Geological Survey – National Water-Quality Assessment (NAWQA) Program. Online. Available HTTP: <http://water.usgs.gov/nawqa/> (accessed: 4 April 2003).
NAWQA provides an assessment of water use in the US and of pesticides in the streams, rivers, and ground water of the United States.

■ California Department of Pesticide Regulation. Online. Available HTTP: <http://www.cdpr.ca.gov/> (accessed: 4 April 2003).
The mission of this Department is "to protect human health and the environment by regulating pesticide sales and use, and by fostering reduced-risk pest management".

### 6.10.4 Non-government organizations

■ Pesticide Action Network North America (PANNA). Online. Available HTTP: <http://www.panna.org> (accessed: 4 April 2003).
"PANNA works to replace pesticide use with ecologically sound and socially just alternatives."

■ Pesticide Action Network International (PANI). Online. Available HTTP: <http://www.pan-international.org/> (accessed: 4 April 2003).
"PANI is a network of over 600 participating nongovernmental organizations, institutions and individuals in over 60 countries working to replace the use of hazardous pesticides with ecologically sound alternatives (English, French, Spanish)."

■ Pesticide Database site – by Pesticide Action Network North America (PAN). Online. Available HTTP: <http://www.pesticideinfo.org/> (accessed: 4 April 2003).
"The PAN Pesticide Database brings together a diverse array of information on pesticides from many different sources, providing human toxicity (chronic and acute), ecotoxicity and regulatory information for about 5400 pesticide active ingredients and their transformation products, as well as adjuvants and solvents used in pesticide products."

■ National Pesticide Telecommunications Network (NPTN). Online. Available HTTP: <http://ace.orst.edu/info/nptn/> (accessed: 4 April 2003).
NPTN is based at Oregon State University and is cooperatively sponsored by the University and EPA. NPTN serves as a source of objective, science-based pesticide information on a wide range of pesticide-related topics, such as recognition and management of pesticide poisonings, safety information, health and environmental effects, referrals for investigation of pesticide incidents and emergency treatment for both humans and animals, and cleanup and disposal procedures.

- Beyond Pesticides. Online. Available HTTP: <http://www.beyondpesticides. org/> (accessed: 4 April 2003).
  "Beyond Pesticides is a national network committed to pesticide safety and the adoption of alternative pest management strategies which reduce or eliminate a dependency on toxic chemicals."
- EXTOXNET InfoBase. Online. Available HTTP: <http://ace.orst.edu/info/ extoxnet/> (accessed: 4 April 2003).
  EXTOXNET provides a variety of information about pesticides, including: the Pesticide Information Profiles (PIPs) for specific information on pesticides and the Toxicology Information Briefs (TIBs) that contain a discussion of certain concepts in toxicology and environmental chemistry.
- Washington Toxics Coalition (WTC). Online. Available HTTP: <www.watoxics.org> (accessed: 4 April 2003).
  WTC provides information on model pesticide policies, alternatives to home pesticides, and much more.
- Monsanto company. Online. Available HTTP: <http://www.monsantoag.com/ monsanto/layout/default.asp> (accessed: 4 April 2003).
  Site contains information on Monsanto company pesticides and agricultural products.

### 6.10.5 References

- MMWR (1999). Farm worker illness following exposure to carbofuran and other pesticides – Fresno County, California, 1998. MMWR, 48(6), 113–116. Online. Available HTTP: <http://www.cdc.gov/mmwr/preview/mmwrhtml/ 00056485.htm> (accessed: 5 July 2003).
- Dean, S. R. and Meola, R. W. (2002). Effect of diet composition on weight gain, sperm transfer, and insemination in the cat flea (Siphonaptera: Pulicidae). J Med Entomol, 39(2), 370–375.
- Dryden, M. W. and Gaafar, S. M. (1991). Blood consumption by the cat flea, *Ctenocephalides felis* (Siphonaptera: Pulicidae). J Med Entomol, 28(3), 394–400.

# Chapter 7

## Lead

## Contents

- Dossier
- Case studies
- Introduction and history
- Biological properties
- Health effects
- Reducing exposure
- Regulatory standards
- Recommendation and conclusions
- More information and references

### 7.1 Dossier

**Name:** lead (Pb)
**Use:** batteries, old paint and previously gasoline, hobbies, solder
**Source:** home, paint, dust, children hands-to-mouth, and workplace
**Recommended daily intake:** none (not essential)
**Absorption:** intestine (50% children, 10% adults), inhalation
**Sensitive individuals:** fetus, children, and women of childbearing age
**Toxicity/symptoms:** developmental and nervous system, lowered IQ, memory and learning difficulties, behavioral problems
**Regulatory facts:** air – 0.5 mg/m$^3$, drinking water 15 µg/l, not allowed in paint or automobile gasoline

> **General facts:** long history of use, major problem in paint of older housing, areas around old smelters can be contaminated
> **Environmental:** global environmental contaminant
> **Recommendations:** avoid, wash hands, wash children's hands and toys

## 7.2 Case studies

In the second century BC, Dioscorides noted, "Lead makes the mind give way". Despite this warning, the seemingly endless uses of lead has repeatedly brought it into daily use and widespread distribution. In modern times, lead was heavily used in paint and as a gasoline additive. The subtle brain damage that even low levels of lead exposure caused in children was recognized and acted upon only in the last 30 years. It is now well documented that even blood levels below 10 μg/dl can harm the developing brain. As the following case studies demonstrate, lead is still a serious concern.

### 7.2.1 Take-home lead – 1998

In 1998 a Californian (MMWR, 2001) mother requested a blood lead level determination for her 18-month-old child. The result was a blood lead level (BLL) of 26 μg/dl, which was well above the Center for Disease Control's (CDC) recommended criterion for clinical case management. It was subsequently found that the father had a BLL of 46 μg/dl, which was above the Occupational Safety and Health Administration (OSHA) requirement that workers with BLLs greater than 40 μg/dl receive additional medical examinations. Further testing found that his 4-month-old daughter had a BLL of 24 μg/dl. This worker was employed in a company that refinished antique furniture, some of which was covered with lead-based paint. Subsequent testing of co-workers found that two refinishers had BLLs of 29 and 54 μg/dl and four carpenters had BLLs of 46, 46, 47, and 56 μg/dl. A child in another family had a BLL of 16 μg/dl. What will be the long-term effects on the intellectual abilities of these children?

### 7.2.2 Lead contaminated town – 2001

The children and families of Herculaneum, Missouri have a lead problem (*New York Times*, 2002), a big lead problem. Herculaneum is home to Doe Run Company, one of the largest lead smelters in the United States, producing 160,000 tons of lead per year. A generation ago, over 800 tons of lead was released into the environment as part of the smelting process. This was reduced to 81 tons in 2001 and the target is 34 tons in 2002. There are signs on the main street informing people about the "high-lead levels on streets" and warning children not to play in the streets or on curbs. A quarter of children under 6 years old were found to have lead poisoning. The US EPA is working to reduce childhood exposure to lead and the company has purchased a number of the most affected homes. How has lead affected the children of Herculaneum? Who is responsible for reducing this hazard?

## 7.3 Introduction and history

> If we were to judge of the interest excited by any medical subject by the number of writings to which it has given birth, we could not but regard the poisoning by lead as the most important to be known of all those that have been treated of, up to the present time.
>
> M. P. Orfila, *A General System of Toxicology*, 1817.

Lead provides many insightful lessons for a student of toxicology, history, and society. During over 8000 years of using lead, we have relearned, forgotten, and ignored lessons on the health effects of lead. Lead is naturally present at very low levels in soil and water prior to the extensive environmental distribution by people, but has no beneficial biological effects. Its physical properties of low melting point, easy malleability, corrosion resistance, and easy availability make it well suited to applications both ancient and modern. It is found alongside gold and silver making lead both a by-product and a contaminant during the smelting of these precious metals. The earliest recorded lead mine dates from 6500 BC in Turkey.

# Pb Lead

## Atomic number: 82
## Atomic mass 207.20

Significant production of lead began about 3000 BC and was first widely used by the Roman Empire. Large mines in Spain and Greece contributed to the global atmospheric redistribution of lead. Easily manipulated, lead was used by the Romans in plumbing. In fact, the word plumbing is derived from *plumbum*, Latin for lead, which also gave rise to the chemical symbol for lead, Pb. Lead is slightly sweet to taste, making it a good additive for fine Roman wine that was then shipped all over Europe. Even in these times, there were reports that lead caused severe colic, anemia, and gout. Some historians believe that lead poisoning hastened the fall of the Roman Empire. For thousands of years, Greenland ice has faithfully recorded the rise and fall of lead use by civilizations that came and went.

In more modern times, the durability of lead made it an excellent paint additive, but the sweetness made it a tempting edible item for young children. Childhood lead poisoning was linked to lead-based paints in 1904. Several European countries banned the use of interior lead-based paints in 1909. At one time baby cribs were painted with lead-based paint, which resulted in infant deaths and other illness. In 1922, the League of Nations banned lead-based paint, but the United States declined to adopt this rule. In 1943, a report concluded that children eating lead paint chips could suffer from neurological disorders including behavioral, learning, and intelligence problems. Finally, in 1971, lead-based paint was phased out in the United States with the passage of the Lead-Based Paint Poisoning Prevention Act. Homes built prior to 1978 may have lead-based paint either inside or outside, and homes and apartments built prior to 1950 will very likely have lead-based paint and should be inspected carefully. This is a particularly serious problem for children living in older housing in large cities. A CDC report found that 35% of African-American children living in inner cities with more than 1 million people had blood lead levels greater that 10 μg/dl, which is the CDC action level established in 1991. In the 1990s, the EPA required that information on lead be disclosed when a home or apartment was being sold or rented. In addition, specific training is required for workers removing lead from homes or apartments. Lead-based paint continues to remain a serious problem for many children.

> Therefore, in contrast to popularized reports, there is no persuasive evidence that low level lead exposure is responsible for any neurobehavioral or intelligence defects. In fact, the bulk of the evidence suggests that there is no adverse impact of low level lead exposure.
> International Lead Zinc Research Organization, October 1982.

> Lead poisoning remains the most common and societal devastating environmental disease of young children.
> Public Health Service – L. Sullivan, 1991.

The addition of lead to gasoline is one of the greatest public health failures of the twentieth century. It is a fascinating story of the intersection of big business, government, and societal interests. Tetraethyl lead (TEL) was discovered in 1854 by a German chemist and in 1921 shown to reduce car engine knock by Thomas Midgley of the United States. This was a period of tremendous competition in the automobile industry and growth in the oil, gas, and chemical industries in the United States. A year latter the US Public Health Service issued a warning about the potential hazards associated with lead. In 1923 the Du Pont Corporation began the first large-scale production of TEL and the first workers died from lead exposure. The same year leaded gasoline went on sale in selected regions of the country. During this period Du Pont acquired a 35% ownership of General Motors, and General Motors and Standard Oil formed a joint company, the Ethyl Corporation, to produce TEL. In 1924, five workers died from lead poisoning at the Ethyl facility in New Jersey, although the number affected by lead exposure is unknown. In 1925, sales of TEL were suspended while the US Surgeon General reviewed its safety. The next year, a committee approved the use of TEL in gasoline and sales were immediately resumed. By 1936, 90% of the gasoline sold in the US contained lead, and the Ethyl Corporation was expanding sales in Europe. In the early 1950s, the US Justice Department investigated anticompetitive activities associated with Du Pont, General Motors, Standard Oil, and the Ethyl Corporation. Environmental concerns were highlighted in a 1965 report documenting that high levels of lead in the environment were caused by human use of lead. In 1972, the US EPA gave notice of an intended phase-out of lead in gasoline and was promptly sued by the Ethyl Corporation. Four years later the EPA standards were upheld in court and, in 1980, the National Academy of Science reported that leaded gasoline was the greatest source of environmental lead contamination.

In 1979, the effects of lead on the intellectual development of children were documented in a seminal paper written by Herbert Needleman and others. The fight over phasing out lead from gasoline was far from over when, in 1981, then Vice President George Bush's task force proposed to relax or eliminate the lead phase-out program. The relationship between leaded gasoline and blood lead levels was demonstrated when the EPA reported that blood lead levels declined by 37% in association with a 50% drop in the use of leaded gasoline between 1976 and 1980. Subsequent studies showed a correlation between the increase in gasoline use during the summer and a rise in blood lead levels. By 1986 the primary phase-out of lead from gasoline was completed, but in some areas of the country, such as Washington State, leaded gasoline was available until 1991. The World Bank called for a ban on leaded gasoline in 1996 and the European Union banned leaded gasoline in 2000. We are still living with the decisions made in the 1920s to add lead to gasoline. It is estimated that 7 million tons of lead were released into the atmosphere from gasoline in the United States alone.

Occupational exposure to lead has decreased from the overt cases of death and disability in the 1930s and 1940s, but, as the case studies illustrate, it continues to occur. In the past, painters using lead-based paints suffered from health problems such as wrist and foot drop or as Ben Franklin reported, the "dangles". Lead paint removal from bridges and buildings is now regulated. Radiator repair and battery recycling continue to be sources of lead exposure. Battery recycling facilities in less developed countries are a serious source of work lead exposure and environmental contamination. Public safety officials who train at shooting ranges using lead ammunition may be exposed to elevated levels of lead. Occupational exposure is a potential hazard not only to the adults but also to their children as lead may be brought home on clothing.

Home hobbies or business can also be a source of lead exposure. Lead is commonly used in stained glass, jewelry making, glazes on pottery, painting, soldering, making ammunition, and exposure can occur from stripping paint from furniture or wood work. Lead glazed pottery has caused a number of lead poisonings, particularly when high-acid foods, which leach lead from the glaze, are consumed from the pottery.

At one time canned foods were a significant source of lead because of poor-quality solder joints in the cans. High-acid goods, such as tomatoes, would leach lead from the cans. Finally, contamination of drinking water with lead occurs primarily from lead solder joints or old fixtures and occasionally lead pipe was used to bring water to a home. As with many metals, lead was used in a number of remedies, some of which are still available and used by some ethnic groups.

## 7.4 Biological properties

The absorption, distribution, and subsequent health effects of lead illustrate the basic principles of toxicology. Foremost is the sensitivity of children to the adverse effects of even low levels of lead exposure and second is dose. There are many reasons why children are more sensitive to lead. Children are much smaller than adults and by weight will receive a much higher dose given the same exposure. Differences in absorption of lead also increase the sensitivity of children. Adults absorb only 5–10% of orally ingested lead, while children absorb approximately 50% and can absorb much more depending on their nutrition. Children and pregnant women will absorb more lead because their bodies have a greater demand for calcium and iron, and the intestine responds by favoring their absorption. Lead substitutes for calcium and is thus readily absorbed, particularly if a diet is low in calcium and iron. Children in families of low income are often in older housing that contains lead and with a poor diet are most vulnerable to the developmental effects of lead. The same is true for pregnant women, whose bodies need more calcium.

Lead distributes in several compartments within the body, each with a different half-life. When lead enters the bloodstream it attaches to red blood cells and in the blood has a half-life of about 25 days. Lead readily crosses the placenta, thus exposing the developing fetus and fetal nervous system to lead. Lead is also stored in the muscle, where it has a longer half-life of about 40 days. Calcium requirements for children are high in part because of rapid bone growth. Lead readily substitutes for calcium and is stored in bone, which was actually visible in radiographs of children with very high lead exposure (fortunately this is very rare now, at least in the United States). In normal circumstances, bone turnover or half-life is very long, so the half-life of lead in the bone is about 20 years. However, if bone turnover is increased, the lead in the bone is mobilized into the blood. This can occur during pregnancy or in older women subject to osteoporosis, which can be caused by decreasing estrogen levels. We accumulate lead over a lifetime, but particularly when we are young, so that as adults our bone and teeth contain approximately 95% of the total lead in the body. As we shall see the short half-life of lead in the blood made tooth lead levels an important indicator of childhood lead exposure and a vital marker to use in correlating with developmental effects.

## 7.5 Health effects

> How long a useful truth may be known and exist, befor it is generally receiv'd and practis'd on.
>
> Benjamin Franklin, 1763.

Lead is one of the most intensively studied hazardous compounds of the twentieth century. The more toxicologists and other researchers investigated the health effects of lead, the more they realized that even very low levels of lead exposure were hazardous. The most common biomarker of lead exposure is the blood lead level, usually measured in micrograms ($\mu$g) per one hundredth of a liter of blood (dl) or $\mu$g/dl. For example, many regulatory agencies set 40 $\mu$g/dl as a level of concern for adult male workers. Typically, at this level workers would be removed from the environment responsible for the exposure and ideally some determination would be made as to the cause of the exposure. The blood level of concern for children has dropped steadily, as shown in Figure 7.1.

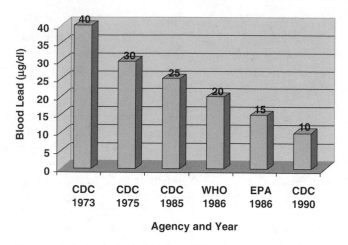

***Figure 7.1.*** Acceptable childhood blood lead levels.

The decline in acceptable childhood blood levels was a function of research and improved control of lead contamination, such as the removal of lead from gasoline. A blood lead level of 10 µg/dl does not represent a "safe" level, only one where it is prudent to take action to reduce exposure. But it must be noted that a level of 10 µg/dl is considered an action level and does not provide any margin of safety for a child's developing nervous system. Currently, there appears to be no safe level of lead exposure for the developing child.

The nervous system is the most sensitive target of lead poisoning. Fetuses and young children are especially vulnerable to the neurological effects of lead because their brains and nervous systems are still developing. At high levels of lead exposure, the brain will swell (encephalopathy), possibly resulting in death. At one time it was thought that children who survived high levels of exposure would recover and lead normal lives. In the 1940s, the persistent learning and developmental effects were demonstrated in children exposed to high levels of lead. In 1979, a study by Needleman showed that even low levels of lead exposure would reduce the school performance of children. This study was one of the first to use tooth lead as a marker of childhood exposure, which correctly classified early childhood exposure even if current blood lead levels were normal. Numerous studies found similar results, and it is now generally accepted that for every 10 µg/dl increase in blood lead levels there is a 2- to 4-point IQ deficit within the range of 5 to 35 µg/dl. While an IQ drop of a few points my not seem like much over the entire population, it is very serious and even more serious for the individuals affected. Subsequent long-term studies of infants and young children exposed to lead showed that as they became older there was an increased likelihood that they would suffer from decreased attention span, reading and learning disabilities, and failure to graduate from high school.

Adult nervous system effects are also apparent following lead exposure. In the past, painters using lead-based paint developed damage to the peripheral nervous system, which caused a wrist or foot drop. Nerve damage can be evaluated in the forearm by using an instrument to measure how fast the nerve conducts an electrical signal from one point to the next. But, as was the case in children, when more subtle effects were looked for, they were found. In adults with blood levels greater that 25 µg/dl there is evidence of decreased cognitive performance.

Lead exposure can produce a number of other effects. One of the most common effects is on the red blood cells, which results in anemia. The red blood cells become fragile and hemoglobin synthesis is impaired. Changes in the red blood cells and some enzymatic changes were used as a marker for lead exposure. Similar to other metals, lead adversely affects kidney function, but this is now rare with reductions in occupational exposure. Several studies have demonstrated that elevated lead exposure is related to elevated blood pressure levels, particularly in men. There appears to be a weak association between lead exposure and increased incidence of lung and brain cancer. Lead exposure is a reproductive hazard for both males and females. In males, lead affects sperm count and sperm motility, resulting in decreased offspring.

The fact that children are more sensitive to the effects of lead exposure is illustrated in Figure 7.2. It is clear that the amount of lead it takes to kill someone is not nearly as important as the lifetime effects on the quality of life.

## 7.6 Reducing exposure

While there are standards for lead exposure, at this time there is no level that is considered safe, so the best policy is to avoid lead exposure. This is difficult because as a contaminant in food, water, or dust, lead cannot be seen, tasted, or smelled. The next best thing is to be aware of potential sources of lead and take appropriate action. For example, if you are moving into an older home with young children or you are planning to start a family, have the paint and soil around the house tested for lead. If the house is old it may contain pipes or solder joints with lead or fixtures with high concentrations of lead. Test kits are available in some stores, but these generally only indicate if lead is present, not how much. Home renovation is an important source of lead exposure. Sanding or removing paint may create dust with high concentrations of lead. Young children exhibit hand-to-mouth behaviors and will ingest significant amounts of lead just from the dust. The EPA has information on safe home renovation.

If you work or come into contact with lead, wash your hands as soon as possible. If you handle lead and then eat, whatever you touch with your hands will contain a small amount of lead. Removing your shoes before coming into the house will reduce carrying in dust that contains lead. This is particularly important if there is an indication of soil contamination such as might occur near or downwind from a smelter. Beware of any hobby or products that might contain lead. Reduce or eliminate lead-based products whenever possible. Most states now ban lead pellets for hunting because the lead pellets are a hazard to birds and contaminate the environment with lead. Old cooking utensils, leaded crystal, and some pottery glaze may contain lead that will leach into foods, particularly those high in acid. Even some cosmetics contain lead, particularly hair coloring products that gradually hide gray hair. Tobacco contains a small amount of lead, another reason to avoid inhalation of tobacco smoke.

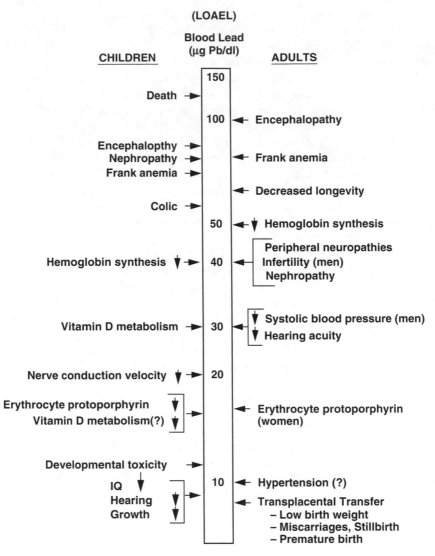

**Figure 7.2.** Effects of lead – children vs adults. Adapted from: ATSDR, 1989, by S. G. Gilbert.

## 7.7 Regulatory standards

Governmental agencies have set limits on lead in the drinking water and in occupational settings. State laws also exist and may be more stringent that the US Federal government.

■   OSHA – lead in air – 0.5 mg/in³ (milligrams per cubic meter)
■   EPA maximum level for lead in public drinking water systems is 15 µg/l

## 7.8 Recommendation and conclusions

The developing nervous system of children is by far the most sensitive to lead exposure. Because of a child's small size and greater absorption of lead, even a very low level of exposure results in a high dose of lead. The developing nervous system is exquisitely sensitive to the effects of even small amounts of lead, resulting in life-long learning deficits. Exposure to lead at an early age clearly deprives a child of his or her ability to express their genetic potential. The optimal action is to avoid lead exposure and ensure children and pregnant women have an adequate diet with appropriate calcium and iron. Additional recommendations include washing your hands and taking off your shoes to reduce dust in the home.

## 7.9 More information and references

### 7.9.1 Slide presentation

■ A Small Dose of Lead presentation material. Online. Available HTTP: <http://www.crcpress.com/e_products/> and follow the links to downloads and then the catalog number TF1691.
Web site contains presentation material related to the health effects of lead.

### 7.9.2 European, Asian, and international agencies

■ International Programme on Chemical Safety (IPCS). Online. Available HTTP: <http://www.who.int/pcs/> (accessed: 4 April 2003).
"The two main roles of the IPCS are to establish the scientific health and environmental risk assessment basis for safe use of chemicals (normative functions) and to strengthen national capabilities for chemical safety (technical cooperation)."

### 7.9.3 North American agencies

■ Health Canada – Lead. Online. Available HTTP: <http://www.hc-sc.gc.ca/english/iyh/environment/lead.html> (accessed: 9 April 2003).
Health Canada provides information on the health effects of lead and remediation programs.
■ US Environmental Protection Agency (EPA) Office of Pollution Prevention and Toxics – Lead Program. Online. Available HTTP: <http://www.epa.gov/opptintr/lead/index.html> (accessed: 4 April 2003).
Site has information on lead health effects and lead abatement.
■ US Centers for Disease Control and Prevention (CDC). Online. Available HTTP: <http://www.cdc.gov/nceh/lead/lead.htm> (accessed: 4 April 2003).
Site has information on CDC lead program.
■ US Department of Housing and Urban Development (HUD) – Office of Healthy Homes and Lead Hazard Control. Online. Available HTTP: <www.hud.gov/offices/lead> (accessed: 4 April 2003).
Site contains information on lead in English and Spanish.

- US EPA Safe Drinking Water Hotline – Phone: 1-800-426-4791
- US Department of Labor Occupational Safety & Health Administration. Online. Available HTTP: <http://www.osha-slc.gov/SLTC/lead/index.html> (accessed: 4 April 2003).
  This site addresses workplace lead exposure.
- US Agency for Toxic Substance Disease Registry (ATSDR). Online. Available HTTP: <http://www.nsc.org/ehc/lead.htm> (accessed: 4 April 2003).
  Toxicology Profile Series – Lead – The Lead Poisoning Prevention Outreach Program funded by the Environmental Health Center (EHC).

### 7.9.4 Non-government organizations

- The National Lead Information Center – Phone: 1-800-424-LEAD (424–5323)
- Alliance To End Childhood Lead Poisoning. Online. Available HTTP: <www.aeclp.org> (accessed: 4 April 2003).
- Washington Swan Working Group – an Affiliate of The Trumpeter Swan Society – Lead Poisoning. Online. Available HTTP:
  <http://www.swansociety.org/issues/lead/0102lead.html> (accessed: 24 April 2003).
  Site has information on the lead poisoning of swans.

### 7.9.5 References

- MMWR (2001) Occupational and take-home lead poisoning associated with restoring chemically stripped furniture – California, 1998. 50(13), 246–248. Online. Available HTTP:
  <http://www.cdc.gov/mmwr/preview/mmwrhtml/mm5013a2.htm> (accessed: 5 July 2003).
- Needleman, H. L. (2000). The removal of lead from petrol: historical and personal reflections. Environ Res. 84(1), 20–35.
- C. H. Rubin, E. Esteban, D. B. Reissman, W. R. Daley, G. P. Noonan, A. Karpati, E. Gurvitch, S. V. Kuzmin, L. I. Privalova, A. Zukov, and A. Zlepko. Lead Poisoning among Young Children in Russia: Concurrent Evaluation of Childhood Lead Exposure in Ekaterinburg, Krasnouralsk, and Volgograd. *Environmental Health Perspectives Volume 110*, Number 6, June 2002
- P. J. Landrigan, C. B. Schechter, J. M. Lipton, M. C. Fahs, and J. Schwartz. Environmental Pollutants and Disease in American Children: Estimates of Morbidity, Mortality, and Costs for Lead Poisoning, Asthma, Cancer, and Developmental Disabilities. *Environmental Health Perspectives Volume 110*, Number 7, July 2002
- D. E. Jacobs, R. P. Clickner, J. Y. Zhou, S. M. Viet, D. A. Marker, J. W. Rogers, D. C. Zeldin, P. Broene, and W. Friedman. The Prevalence of Lead-Based Paint Hazards in US Housing. *Environmental Health Perspectives Volume 110*, Number 10, October 2002

# Chapter 8

# Mercury

## Contents

## 8.1 Dossier – inorganic mercury

**Name:** mercury (Hg) (inorganic)
**Use:** consumer products, industry, dental amalgams, switches, thermometers
**Source:** mining, environment, workplace
**Recommended daily intake:** none (not essential)
**Absorption:** inhalation, intestine poor
**Sensitive individuals:** fetus, children, women of childbearing age
**Toxicity/symptoms:** nervous system, irritability, drowsiness, depression, incoordination, and tremors ("mad as a hatter")

**Regulatory facts:** ATSDR – minimal risk level (MRL) – inhalation 0.2 μg/m$^3$
**General facts:** long history of use, liquid silver evaporates at room temperature, bacteria convert to organic methyl mercury
**Environmental:** global environmental contaminant
**Recommendations:** avoid, recycle mercury-containing devices

## 8.2 Dossier – organic mercury

**Name:** mercury (organic) (methyl mercury – Hg-CH$_3$)
**Use:** limited laboratory use
**Source:** contaminates some fish (e.g. tuna, shark, pike)
**Recommended daily intake:** none (not essential)
**Absorption:** intestine (90%)
**Sensitive individuals:** fetus, children, women of childbearing age
**Toxicity/symptoms:** nervous system, developmental effects include cerebral palsy-like symptoms with involvement of the visual, sensory, and auditory systems, tingling around lips and mouth, tingling in fingers and toes, vision and hearing loss
**Regulatory facts:** EPA – RfD – 0.1 μg/kg per day
FDA – 1 ppm in commercial fish
ATSDR – MRL – 0.30 μg/kg per day
**General facts:** bacteria convert inorganic mercury to methyl mercury, then it enters the food chain (bioaccumulation)
**Environmental:** global environmental contaminant, bioaccumulates in some fish
**Recommendations:** avoid, recycle mercury-containing devices

## 8.3 Case studies

### 8.3.1 Minamata, Japan – mercury and fish

In the late 1950s the subtle and serious consequences of methyl mercury exposure became evident in Minamata, Japan. Initially, early signs of uncoordinated movement and numbness around the lips and extremities, followed by constriction in visual fields in fishermen and their families, baffled health experts. Developmental effects were clearly evident in infants who exhibited subtle to severe disabilities. This spectrum of adverse effects was finally related to methyl mercury exposure from consumption of contaminated fish. Minamata Bay was contaminated with mercury and methyl mercury from a factory manufacturing the chemical acetaldehyde. Mercury was used in the manufacturing process, which also resulted in both mercury and methyl mercury being discharged into Minamata Bay. The fish in the bay accumulated increasing amounts of methyl mercury, which was subsequently passed to the fish-consuming residents of the area. This was one of the first modern lessons of the consequences of the bioaccumulation of methyl mercury.

### 8.3.2 Mercury and gold mining

Environmental contamination from the use of mercury in gold mining started centuries ago and continues today. The Peruvian Incas first used elemental mercury in gold mining in the 1500s. The gold binds to the mercury, and when the mercury is removed the gold is left behind. Imagine heating a pan of a silvery substance (mercury–gold amalgam) and watching it turn to gold, a trick worthy of any alchemist. The mercury literally evaporates into the atmosphere leaving the gold behind. This practice continues today in Central and South America, Africa, and the Philippines. It is estimated that it takes approximately 3 to 5 kg of mercury to extract 1 kg of gold. A large portion of this mercury contaminates the local environment, and by moving into the atmosphere, can be rained down to earth many miles and even countries away, contributing to the global mercury contamination. The elemental mercury is converted to methyl mercury by bacteria after which it moves up the food chain, often in fish that are consumed by a range of animals and humans. Local miners, their families, and particularly children suffer from mercury exposure.

### 8.3.3 Mercury-coated seed grain in Iraq

The toxic antifungal properties of organic mercury compounds were found to be beneficial when applied to seed grain, but when humans consumed these seeds there were tragic consequences. During much of the twentieth century, seeds were coated with organomercury compounds to reduce their destruction by fungus in the soil. Often these seeds were pink colored to indicate they were coated with an antifungal agent and were for planting only, not consumption. During the early 1970s, a severe drought in Iraq resulted in a loss of seed grain as people struggled with malnutrition. Pink-colored mercury-coated seed grain was shipped to Iraq for planting. Unfortunately, the local population could not read the foreign language on the seed bags nor recognize the pink seeds as hazardous. Bread made from these seeds was pink, tasty, and toxic, particularly to the developing child. Many people died or were tragically disabled for life, giving the world another lesson in communication and mercury toxicity.

### 8.3.4 Mercury in paint

Prior to the 1990s mercury compounds were routinely added to interior and exterior paint to prevent bacterial and fungal growth. The practice of adding mercury to paint was halted after the adverse effects of inhaled mercury were seen in a 4-year-old boy. The child's unventilated bedroom was painted with mercury-containing interior latex paint. The boy was diagnosed with acrodynia; a rare disease caused by mercury exposure and characterized by flushed cheeks, pink, scaling palms and toes, profuse sweating, insomnia, and irritability. Manufacturers agreed to discontinue the use of mercury in paint in 1991, but because people often store paint for long periods of time, this existing paint could still cause health problems (MMWR, 1996a).

### 8.3.5 Mercury under floorboards

Mercury is commonly used in many industrial applications and is a source of a nasty surprise when not adequately removed. In 1996 it was reported that six children and a number of adults were exposed to mercury vapor while living in condominiums in a converted manufacturing building. Prior to being converted, this building had been used to manufacture mercury vapor lamps. Pools of mercury were discovered beneath the floorboards of the condominiums.

## 8.4 Introduction and history

Mercury exists in different forms with very different properties; thus each section of this chapter is divided into inorganic mercury – the common silvery liquid – and organic mercury (usually methyl mercury – $Hg-CH_3$) that is generated from mercury and accumulates in some commonly consumed species of fish.

Mercury's dual nature of being both industrially useful and potentially harmful was recognized historically, but only in the last 20 years have we begun to appreciate its more subtle qualities and effects. The contradictory nature of mercury was recognized in Roman mythology, in which the winged messenger Mercury, who was noted for his cleverness, cunning, and eloquence, was both the god of merchants and commerce as well as thieves and vagabonds. The history of mercury's use by humans shows our struggle to balance and understand the usefulness of this compound and its harmful effects to humans and the environment. We now grapple with mercury as a global pollutant as we recognize its potential risks to children.

> For then she bore a son, of many shifts, blandly cunning, a robber, a cattle driver, a bringer of dreams, a watcher by night, a thief at the gates, one who was soon to show forth wonderful deeds among the deathless gods . . .
>
> Description of the birth of the Greek god Mercury.

### 8.4.1 Inorganic mercury

Elemental mercury, also known as quicksilver or metallic mercury, is a silvery liquid at room temperature, with a low boiling point, a high vapor pressure (e.g. evaporates) at room temperature, and a high density, weighing 13.6 times as much as water. Stone, iron, lead, and even humans can float on its surface (see Putman, 1972). Its toxicity has been recognized since Roman times when slaves mined it in Almaden, Spain; this mine remains active today as a major mercury source. While all rock types contain some mercury, cinnabar contains the greatest concentration of inorganic mercury (>80%). Elemental mercury is produced from cinnabar by condensing the vapor of heated ore. In the United States elemental mercury is produced primarily as a byproduct of mining.

# Hg Mercury

## Atomic Number: 80
## Atomic Mass: 200

Elemental mercury is used industrially in electric lamps and switches, gauges and controls (e.g. thermometers, barometers, thermostats), battery production, nuclear weapons production, and the specialty chemical industry, including the production of caustic soda. Because elemental mercury has a high affinity for gold and silver, it has been, and continues to be, used in precious metal extraction from ore. Elemental mercury has been used for over one hundred years in mercury–silver amalgam preparations to repair dental caries. Mercury continues to be used in folk remedies and in certain cultural practices, with unknown public health implications.

The Chinese used cinnabar to make red ink before 1000 BC, and in cosmetics, soaps, and laxatives. Inorganic mercury (as an acid of mercury nitrate) was used in the felting industry to aid in matting felt; felting was a leading source of occupational mercury exposure in the United States into the 1940s. A 1937 Census of Manufacture of the US Census Bureau reported 5.2 million pounds of hatter's fur used in the production of over 30 million felt-hat bodies among 140 factories in the United States, and a study of 25 Connecticut hat factories demonstrated evidence of chronic mercurialism among 59 of 534 hatters.

Peruvian Incas used elemental mercury to wash gold-bearing gravel as early as 1557. The original extraction process, which took place over 20 to 30 days, underwent subsequent modification, leading to the ability to extract gold in a pan over a fire in less than 6 hours by the 1830s. With some modifications this process continues to be used to this day, especially in Central and South America, Africa, and the Philippines.

Dental amalgams were used as early as the seventh century, and the first commercial mercury dental amalgam was used in the 1830s in New York. Chronic mercury exposure among dentists and dental assistants is a well-recognized occupational hazard. Concerns over the public health risks of mercury amalgam fillings have also been raised in the scientific literature, though this is an area of significant controversy. Recent studies indicate that the amount of mercury in urine is related to the number of dental amalgams and that a similar relationship exists for mercury excretion in human breast milk.

> Wipe off this glass three times.
> There is arsenic in it.
> I hear messages from God
> through the fillings in my teeth.
> Anne Sexton (1928–1974).

Mercury thermometers have been used for decades. In some instances their use has been discontinued, such as in infant incubators where it was found that significant mercury vapor concentrations could be achieved if the thermometers were broken in this enclosed environment. Disposal of thermometers and thermostats continues to add significantly to the toxicity of municipal waste. In 1995, discarded thermometers contributed 16.9 tons of mercury to municipal solid waste stream.

### 8.4.2 Organic mercury

The first reported use of organic mercury compounds in chemical research occurred in 1863. Their synthesis immediately led to the recognition of their extremely high toxicity relative to inorganic mercury forms, and by 1866 two chemists had died from organic mercury poisoning. Therapeutic applications of organic mercurials in the treatment of central nervous system syphilis, which began in 1887, led to non-occupational poisoning; the use of organic mercury-based medicines ceased soon after because of their extremely high toxicity. The use of synthetic organic mercurials as antifungal dressings for agricultural seeds began in 1914. Their use in this industry has resulted in scattered case reports of acute poisoning associated with the chemical manufacture, application, and inadvertent consumption of either the treated grain or of animals fed with the treated grain. The use of organic mercurials in agriculture has resulted in large-scale poisoning episodes worldwide, such as occurred in Iraq.

Both elemental mercury and inorganic mercury are used in chemical manufacture, including vinyl chloride and acetaldehyde synthesis (inorganic mercury), and chlor-alkali production (elemental mercury). For example, the Minamata factory used mercuric oxide dissolved in sulfuric acid as a catalyst for the hydration of acetylene to acetaldehyde. In addition, vinyl chloride production at the Minamata factory used mercuric chloride absorbed on to activated carbon for the production of vinyl chloride from acetylene and hydrogen chloride. It is these processes that directly led to the contamination of Minamata Bay and the Agano River, and Niigata by mercury effluent. This discharge resulted in large-scale human methyl mercury exposure and toxicity during the 1950s and 1960s, and led to our present-day appreciation of mercury's environmental cycling, biomethylation, and food chain transfer.

Organic mercury compounds have also been used in latex paint to extend the shelf life, though such uses are currently restricted in the United States following the recognition of this potential hazard to children. Subsequent evaluation of interior rooms of homes painted with mercury-containing latex paint found that mercury vapor concentrations were elevated and in several cases were above the $0.5 \ \mu g/m^3$ concentration recommended by the Agency for Toxic Substances and Disease Registry.

## 8.5 Biological properties

### 8.5.1 Inorganic mercury

Inorganic mercury can also be in the form of salts as either monovalent ($Hg^+$, mercuric) or divalent ($Hg^{2+}$, mercurous). Two major mercury chloride salts, calomel

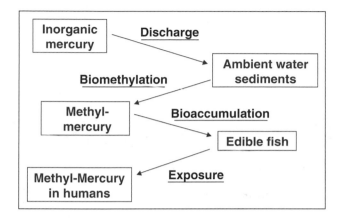

**Figure 8.1.** Mercury to methyl mercury.

(mercurous chloride) and sublimate (mercuric chloride) were first produced in the Middle Ages. Inorganic mercury-based skin creams were first used during this period for the treatment of syphilis, and inorganic mercury was used as a clinical diuretic during the early 1900s. When mercury vapor from elemental mercury is inhaled, it is readily and rapidly absorbed into the bloodstream, and easily crosses the blood–brain barrier and the placenta. Ingestion of elemental mercury is far less hazardous than inhalation of mercury vapor due to its poor absorption in the gut. After entering the brain, mercury is oxidized and will not transfer back across the blood–brain barrier, thus continued exposure to mercury vapor will result in mercury accumulation in the nervous system.

### 8.5.2 Organic mercury

While there are many synthetic organic mercury compounds, the most important organic mercury is the naturally occurring form methyl mercury (MeHg). In the environment, inorganic mercury is biotransformed to MeHg primarily through microbial methylation in sediments of fresh and sea waters (Figure 8.1). Once produced, MeHg readily enters the aquatic food chain and bioaccumulates in tissues of aquatic organisms. Because MeHg is stored throughout the life of aquatic organisms, it is transferred up the food chain and results in the highest concentrations in larger, long-lived, predatory species such as swordfish, pike, and ocean tuna. The bulk of mercury in fish is stored in muscle, and almost all of the mercury in muscle is MeHg. The concentration of MeHg in fish depends on the age and trophic level of the particular fish, and can be quite substantial (> 1000 μg/kg (ppm)). For example, the total mercury in the edible tissues of shark and swordfish can average as high as 1200 μg/kg. Organomercurials have been used as fungicides, as paint preservatives, and in medicinal applications, though these uses have ceased as a result of their recognized neurotoxicity. Therefore, fish and marine mammal consumption are the primary sources of human MeHg exposure, and to a lesser degree research applications of MeHg and other organomercurials.

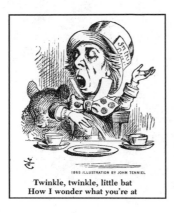

Twinkle, twinkle, little bat
How I wonder what you're at

**Figure 8.2.** The Mad Hatter.

## 8.6 Health effects

### 8.6.1 Inorganic mercury

Elemental mercury in the form of mercury vapor is readily and rapidly absorbed into the bloodstream when inhaled and easily crosses the blood–brain barrier and the placenta. Oral ingestion of elemental mercury is far less hazardous than inhalation of mercury vapor due to its poor absorption in the gut. Acute, high level exposure to mercury vapor can result in respiratory, cardiovascular, neurological, and gastrointestinal effects, and even death.

Either acute, high-dose or chronic, low-dose exposure to mercury vapor can result in increasing and irreversible neurological effects. Symptoms include tremors and loss of feeling in the hands (paresthesia or stocking-glove sensory loss), emotional instability, insomnia, memory loss, and neuromuscular weakness. Exposure to mercury vapor may precipitate tremor, drowsiness, depression, and irritability; such symptoms form the basis for the expression "mad as a hatter" and the Mad Hatter in Lewis Carroll's, *Alice's Adventures in Wonderland*. (Figure 8.2). Decreased performance on memory tests and verbal concept formation has also been documented in industry workers exposed to mercury vapor. Neurotoxic effects such as dizziness, weakness, insomnia, numbness, and tremor were observed in a 12-year-old girl exposed to spilled mercury.

### 8.6.2 Organic mercury

The devastating health consequences of methyl mercury (MeHg) exposure were well documented from several tragic incidents (see the case studies section). Historically, MeHg exposure played a very important role in drawing worldwide attention to the consequences of industrial pollution, not just for workers but also for the general public. In the 1950s, the consequences of MeHg exposure to the people of Minamata and Niigata, Japan were recognized. In both cases MeHg exposure resulted from consumption of fish from waters receiving industrial effluent discharge

### Table 8.1 Major mercury poisoning incidents

| Place | Year | Cases |
|---|---|---|
| Minamata | 1953–60 | 1,000 |
| Niigata | 1964–65 | 646 |
| Guatemala | 1963–65 | 45 |
| Ghana | 1967 | 144 |
| Pakistan | 1969 | 100 |
| Iraq | 1956 | 100 |
| Iraq | 1960 | 1,002 |
| Iraq | 1971 | 40,000 |
| Ongoing | 2001 | ??? |

containing mercurials, which demonstrated conclusively that MeHg poisoning could occur through food-chain transfer of MeHg. By 1974, over 2150 cases of, what was as then called, Minamata disease had been established in the Minamata region alone. Observations of an abnormally high incidence of cerebral palsy-like symptoms with involvement of the visual, sensory, and auditory systems among children from the Minamata region also heralded a new concern over the potential developmental toxicity of industrially derived MeHg. However, as with the adult cases of MeHg poisoning, a causal relationship between environmental MeHg and cases of observed infantile developmental toxicity was difficult to establish. Difficulties in making an association arose because the affected children had not eaten fish and there were no identified neurological effects in their mothers based on evaluations at that time. The susceptibility and the sensitivity of the fetus, relative to adults, to MeHg-induced neurotoxicity were later documented in other studies.

A tragic incident in Iraq clearly documented the fetal effects of maternal methyl mercury exposure (see case study section). During the winter of 1971, some 73,000 tons of wheat and 22,000 tons of barley were imported into Iraq. This grain, intended for planting, was treated with various organic mercurials. Unfortunately, this grain was made into flour and consumed throughout the country, resulting in the hospitalization of some 6530 people and death of 459 at the time of the study (Table 8.1).

The accumulated evidence leaves no doubt that MeHg is a serious developmental toxicant in humans, especially to the nervous system. While the toxicological, and behavioral outcomes resulting from high-concentration *in utero* MeHg exposures are not in debate, questions regarding risks and mechanisms of action following low-concentration, chronic *in utero* exposures remain.

A US National Research Council report states "over 60,000 newborns annually might be at risk for adverse neurodevelopmental effects from *in utero* exposure to MeHg (methyl mercury)". This report clearly makes the point that many infants are exposed to mercury above levels considered safe.

One of the complications with diagnosing MeHg exposure is that presentation of symptoms appears to occur after a latency period during which no effects are observed. The period of latency appears to be related to the level of exposure, with higher exposure concentrations resulting in a shorter latency period. The exact biological mechanisms underlying this latency period are unclear. Some researchers have suggested that latency not only reflects the time to reach accumulation of MeHg in the brain, but also reflects achievement of a threshold wherein enough tissue is destroyed so that the capacity of the central nervous system to compensate for the damage is overwhelmed. Observation of long latencies following cessation of MeHg administration in animals and humans, however, may also derive from long-term demethylation of MeHg to inorganic mercury in the brain.

## 8.7 Reducing exposure

### 8.7.1 Inorganic mercury

There are numerous sources of metallic mercury in the home and workplace. The best advice is to dispose properly of any product with mercury and above all avoid exposure, especially inhalation, particularly for young children. In the past few years, many industries have worked to reduce the use of mercury in products. In addition, some states have also restricted the use of mercury or have developed programs to aid in the recycling and recovery of mercury. The average household fever thermometer contains about 3 grams of mercury, which does not seem like much, until it is multiplied by the 105 million households in the United States. Even if only half of the households had a mercury thermometer, the total amount of mercury is very large. Additional sources of atmospheric mercury include coal-fueled electric generation facilities, hospital waste, fluorescent light bulbs, dental surgeries, and even crematoriums. Efforts are being made on a number of fronts to mandate reduction in mercury released into the atmosphere and in general reduce the use of mercury. As individuals, we must also work to ensure mercury products are properly recycled and take action to reduce atmospheric mercury.

If a mercury spill occurs, it is very important to ventilate the area and *not* use a vacuum cleaner to clean up the mercury. A vacuum cleaner will only warm and disperse the mercury in the room. Collect all the mercury and place in a sealed container and take it to an appropriate disposal site. If it is a large spill, professionals must be called. Table 8.2 lists some of the more common sources of metallic mercury.

### 8.7.2 Organic mercury

The primary concern with organic mercury is methyl mercury in fish. Children and women of childbearing age should be cautious about consuming fish known to accumulate mercury such as tuna, shark, swordfish, and pike. Local fish consumption advisories should be followed.

## 8.8 Regulatory standards

### 8.8.1 Inorganic mercury

The liquid silver inorganic mercury evaporates into the atmosphere. When inhaled, mercury crosses easily into the blood and then to the brain, thus the primary

| *Table 8.2* Common sources of metallic mercury |
| --- |

Switches in gas furnaces, heaters, etc.

Major household appliances (tilt switches in freezers, dryers, etc.)

Irons (tilt switches)

Automobile switches

Bilge pumps, sump pumps, etc. (float switches)

Dental amalgam

Measuring devices and laboratory equipment, such as barometers, manometers, etc.

Medical equipment and supplies

Fluorescent lights

Batteries

Computers

Novelty items

Film pack batteries

hazard concern is from inhalation. Metallic mercury is poorly absorbed after oral ingestion, thus this is much less hazardous than inhalation. Below are some of the advisories on mercury vapor inhalation.

- ATSDR – minimal risk level (MRL) – 0.2 $\mu g/m^3$
- OSHA – permissible exposure limits (PEL)-TWA – 0.05 $mg/m^3$
- ACGIH – threshold limit value (TLV)-TWA – 0.05 $mg/m^3$

## 8.8.2 Organic methyl mercury

The primary human exposure to methyl mercury is from consumption of contaminated fish. The most sensitive population is the developing fetus or infant due to the effects of methyl mercury on the nervous system (neurotoxic) and developmental effects. Exposure limits and fish consumption advisories are directed at pregnant women, women of childbearing age, and children. All agencies also recognize that fish consumption has many nutritional benefits and is an important part of many people's diet. Nevertheless, the widespread distribution of mercury and subsequent bioaccumulation of methyl mercury requires that many agencies have developed recommendation for levels of mercury in fish. Below is a list of some of these recommendations, but it is very important to consult the local fish consumption advisories.

- FDA – 1 ppm in commercially harvested fish (i.e. tuna fish)
- FDA – action level – 0.47 $\mu g/kg$ per day
- ATSDR – minimal risk levels (MRLs) – 0.30 $\mu g/kg$ per day
- Washington State – total daily intake – 0.035–0.08 $\mu g/kg$ per day
- EPA – Reference Dose (RfD) – 0.1 $\mu g/kg$ per day
  (In 1997 the EPA estimated that 7% of the women of childbearing age in the United States exceed the established RfD of 0.1 $\mu g/kg$ per day.)
- 41 states have issued over 2000 fish consumption advisories related to mercury

Recommendation from the State of Washington (US)

■  Women of childbearing age should limit the amount of canned tuna they
   eat to about one can per week (six ounces.) A woman who weighs less
   than 135 pounds should eat less than one can of tuna per week.
■  Children under six should eat less than one half a can of tuna (three ounces)
   per week. Specific weekly limits for children under six range from one ounce
   for a twenty pound child, to three ounces for a child weighing about sixty pounds.

See: http://www.doh.wa.gov/fish/FishAdvMercury.htm

## 8.9 Recommendation and conclusions

Mercury is a potent toxicant and a global environmental pollutant. There is over-
whelming data that demonstrate that low levels of exposure to methyl mercury or
mercury vapor damage the nervous system, particularly the sensitive developing nervous system. Mercury vapor travels around the globe in the atmosphere. Once on
the ground or in the water, it is converted to methyl mercury and accumulates in
the food supply, contaminating fish, a main source of protein for many people. There
needs to be a global effort to reduce human release of mercury into the environment. The production, sale, and use of mercury must be restricted in recognition
of the health effects of mercury. Mercury use in consumer products, such as thermostats, thermometers, and jewelry should be eliminated and replaced with already
well-established and cost-effective alternatives. Coal contains low levels of mercury that are released as the coal is burned. The discharge from coal-fired electric
generating facilities can be greatly reduced with current technology. Finally there
must be ongoing monitoring of mercury contamination in fish and appropriate
advisories issued to protect sensitive populations. This will involve education of
the consumer about limiting the consumption of fish that accumulate mercury.

Summary of recommendations on mercury

■  Reduce global environmental release
■  Restrict global production and sale and use
■  Clean up contaminated sites
■  Reduce mercury emission from coal-fired electric power facilities
■  Reduce or eliminate use in consumer products (cars, thermometers, ther-
   mostats, jewelry)
■  Advise women of childbearing age on fish consumption
■  Monitor mercury levels in fish

## 8.10 More information and references

### 8.10.1 Slide presentation

- A Small Dose of Mercury presentation material. Online. Available HTTP: <http://www.crcpress.com/e_products/> and follow the links to downloads and then the catalog number TF1691.
  Web site contains presentation material related to health effects of mercury.

### 8.10.2 European, Asian, and international agencies

- United Nations Environment Program's Global Mercury Assessment. Online. Available HTTP: <http://www.chem.unep.ch/mercury/> (accessed: 5 April 2003).
  This program aims to develop a global assessment of mercury and its compounds, including an outline of options for addressing any significant global adverse impacts of mercury.
- World Health Organization – Mercury. Online. Available HTTP: <http://www.who.int/pcs/cicad/full_text/cicad50.pdf (accessed: 5 April 2003).
  Document on the health effects of organic and inorganic mercury.

### 8.10.3 North American agencies

- Health Canada – Mercury. Online. Available HTTP: <http://www.hc-sc.gc.ca/english/iyh/environment/mercury.html> (accessed: 9 April 2003).
  Health Canada provides information on the health effects and environmental distribution of mercury.
- US Food and Drug Administration (FDA) – Advisory on Methyl Mercury and Fish. Online. Available HTTP: <http://www.cfsan.fda.gov/~lrd/tphgfish.html> (accessed: 5 April 2003).
  Site has recent FDA consumer information on methyl mercury.
- US Environmental Protection Agency (EPA):
  1. EPA – Main site on Mercury. Online. Available HTTP: <http://www.epa.gov/mercury/> (accessed: 5 April 2003).
  2. EPA Advice on Eating Non Commercial Fish – Advice for Women and Children. Online. Available HTTP: <http://www.epa.gov/waterscience/fishadvice/advice.html> (accessed: 5 April 2003).
  3. EPA Fact Sheet: Fish Caught by Family and Friends – Advice for Women and Children. Online. Available HTTP: <http://www.epa.gov/waterscience/fishadvice/factsheet.html> (accessed: 5 April 2003).
  4. EPA (1997). Mercury Study Report to Congress. Office of Air Quality Planning and Standards and Office of Research and Development. EPA-452-R-97 –003 through –010 (Volumes I–VIII0. Online. Available HTTP: <http://www.epa.gov/oar/mercury.html> (accessed: 5 April 2003).
  5. EPA Integrated Risk Information System. Online. Available HTTP: <http://www.epa.gov/iris/index.html>

- US Agency for Toxic Substance Disease Registry (ATSDR) – Toxicology Profile Series on Mercury. Online. Available HTTP: <http://www.atsdr.cdc.gov/toxprofiles/tp46.html> (accessed: 5 April 2003).
  ATSDR produces toxicology profile documents on many compounds including mercury.
- US Agency for Toxic Substance Disease Registry (ATSDR) – Toxicology Profile Series on Mercury. Online. Available HTTP: <http://www.atsdr.cdc.gov/mrls.html> (accessed: 5 April 2003).
  ATSDR's list of minimal risk levels.
- US Department of Labor – Occupational Safety & Health Administration (OSHA). Online. Available HTTP: <http://www.osha.gov/> (accessed: 5 April 2003).
- US Geological Survey (USGS). Online. Available HTTP: <http://www.usgs.gov/> (accessed: 5 April 2003).
  Site has maps and supply information on mercury.
- US National Research Council (NRC) – Toxicological Effects of Methylmercury. Online. Available HTTP: <http://www.nationalacademies.org/publications/> (accessed: 5 April 2003).
  The full NRC report on mercury can be read on the web.
- Washington State Department of Health – Fish Facts for Health Nutrition. Online. Available HTTP: <http://www.doh.wa.gov/fish/> (accessed: 5 April 2003).
  Site has information on Washington State's advisory of fish consumption and mercury.

### 8.10.4 Non-government organizations

- The Mercury Policy Project (MPP). Online. Available HTTP: <http://www.mercurypolicy.org/> (accessed: 5 April 2003).
  "MPP works to raise awareness about the threat of mercury contamination and promote policies to eliminate mercury uses, reduce the export and trafficking of mercury, and significantly reduce mercury exposures at the local, national, and international levels."
- American Conference of Governmental Industrial Hygienists (ACGIH®). Online. Available HTTP: <http://www.acgih.org/home.htm> (accessed: 5 April 2003).
  "ACGIH is a member-based organization and community of professionals that advances worker health and safety through education and the development and dissemination of scientific and technical knowledge."

### 8.10.5 References

- Clarkson, T. (1998). Methylmercury and fish consumption: Weighing the risks. Can Med Assoc J, 158, 1465–1466.
- Clarkson, T. W. (2002). The three modern faces of mercury. Environ Health Perspect, 110 Suppl 1, 11–23.

■ Gilbert, S. G. and Grant-Webster, K. S. (1995). Neurobehavioral effects of developmental methylmercury exposure. Environ Health Perspect, 6, 135–142.

■ Kales, S. N. and Goldman, R. H. (2002). Mercury exposure: current concepts, controversies, and a clinic's experience. J Occup Environ Med, 44(2), 143–154.

■ Martin, D. M., DeRouen, T. A. and Leroux, B. G. (1997). Is mercury amalgam safe for dental fillings? Washington Public Health, 15(Fall), 30–32.

■ MMWR. (1996a). Mercury exposure among residents of a building formerly used for industrial purposes – New Jersey, 1995. Morbidity Mortality Weekly Report, 45(20), 422–424. Online. Available HTTP: <http://www.cdc.gov/mmwr/preview/mmwrhtml/00041880.htm> (accessed: 5 July 2003).

■ MMWR. (1996b). Mercury poisoning associated with beauty cream – Arizona, California, New Mexico and Texas, 1996. Morbidity Mortality Weekly Report, 45(29), 633–635. Online. Available HTTP: <http://www.cdc.gov/mmwr/preview/mmwrhtml/00043182.htm> (accessed: 5 July 2003).

■ Putman J. (1972). Quicksilver and slow death. National Geographic 142(4), 507–527.

■ Zeitz, P., Orr, M. F. and Kaye, W. E. (2002). Public health consequences of mercury spills: Hazardous Substances Emergency Events Surveillance system, 1993–1998. Environ Health Perspect, 110(2), 129–132.

# Chapter 9

# Arsenic

## Contents

### 9.1 Dossier

**Name:** arsenic

**Use:** wood preservative, pesticides, semiconductor manufacturing

**Source:** coal combustion, drinking water, environment, medical drug, seafood

**Recommended daily intake:** none (not essential)

**Absorption:** inhalation, intestine – inorganic high, organic low, skin

**Sensitive individuals:** children

**Toxicity/symptoms:** Peripheral nervous system (tingling in hands and feet), skin cancer (ingestion), lung cancer (inhalation); hyperpigmentation (keratosis) of palms and soles; vascular complications

> **Regulatory facts:** EPA – Drinking water 10 µg/l (0.01 ppm)
> EPA – RfD – 0.3 µg/kg per day
> OSHA – Workplace air 10 µg/m$^3$
> ATSDR – MRL – 0.3 µg/kg per day
> **General facts:** long history of use as medicine and poison
> **Environmental:** global environmental contaminant, bioaccumulates in fish and shellfish (mostly in a form that is not harmful)
> **Recommendations:** avoid, do not use arsenic-treated lumber, test drinking water

## 9.2 Case studies

... (Henry Adams) he found himself invariably taking for granted, as a political instinct, with out waiting further experiment, – as he took for granted that arsenic poisoned, – the rule that a friend in power is a friend lost.
　　　Henry Adams (1838–1918). *The Education of Henry Adams*, 1918.

### 9.2.1 Arsenic in drinking water

Arsenic in drinking water is a worldwide problem affecting the lives of millions of people. High levels of arsenic in local soil or rock contaminate the local water supply. In the United States, the federal government has struggled for many years to establish standards of arsenic in the drinking water. The US Environmental Protection Agency has recently lowered the standard from 50 ppm (50 µg/l) to 10 ppm. This standard will require additional treatment of a number of municipal water supplies, particularly in western United States (see map in presentation). The standard is being lowered because chronic exposure to low levels of arsenic can cause skin cancer and others illnesses. Even at the new standard of 10 ppm, there is a risk of cancer.

In other areas of the world, such as Bangladesh, elevated arsenic levels in the drinking water are more acutely life threatening. People were encouraged to establish local wells to reduce exposure to drinking water contaminated with bacteria. It was subsequently discovered that many of these wells have high levels of arsenic in the water. It is estimated that 75 million people in Bangladesh are exposed to arsenic-contaminated water and that will result in 200,000 to 270,000 deaths from cancer each year. In addition, people suffer from skin changes on the palms of hands and soles of feet (for additional information see presentation).

### 9.2.2 Pressure-treated wood

By far the largest use of arsenic is in treating wood to prevent decay or insect damage. Several compounds are used, but the vast majority of wood is treated with a pesticide called chromated copper arsenate (CCA). CCA is a water-based mixture of inorganic salts of chromium, copper, and arsenic that is forced into the wood under pressure. Wood treated with CCA is used in decks, playground equipment, outdoor furniture, fences, construction lumber, utility poles, piers, and pilings. The amount of arsenic in treated wood can be quite large. A standard eight-foot length of 2 × 4 inch lumber contains as much as 15 grams of arsenic.

The health risks of exposure to arsenic-treated lumber have been debated for years, although it is well known that inhaling sawdust from construction with treated lumber can be quite dangerous. Ideally the arsenic-based wood preservative is "fixed" to the wood, but research has shown that arsenic leaches from the wood with rainfall and arsenic can be rubbed off from the surface by hand contact. Arsenic contamination of soil under decks often exceeds hazardous waste clean-up standards. Children who play on decks or other treated surfaces pick up arsenic on their hands and later ingest some of the arsenic when they put their hands in their mouth or pick up food. Health professionals, the wood preserving industry, and public interest groups have hotly debated the hazards of these exposures. In 2002, producers of arsenic-treated wood reached an agreement with the EPA to phase out the residential uses of arsenic-treated lumber, including decks, play equipment, fences, etc. CCA will still be available for commercial uses such as utility poles. The alternative wood treatment most likely to replace CCA is a copper-based preservative called ammoniacal copper quaternary, or ACQ. ACQ has a much lower toxicity to humans than CCA.

## 9.3 Introduction and history

> I pray my companion, if he wishes for bread, to ask me for bread, and if he wishes for sassafras or arsenic, to ask me for them, and not to hold out his plate, as if I knew already.
>
> Ralph Waldo Emerson (1803–1882).

People long ago recognized that, depending on the dose, arsenic could either treat an illness or be used as a poison to cause death. Its medicinal use to treat syphilis and amebic dysentery ended with the introduction of penicillin and other antibiotics in the twentieth century. Arsenic-based compounds are currently used to treat some forms of cancer. As a poison, arsenic trioxide ($As_2O_3$) has several desirable qualities: it looks like sugar, it is tasteless, and it only takes about a tenth of gram to kill some-

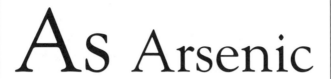

As Arsenic
Atomic Number: 33
Atomic Mass: 74.92

one. While its use as a human poison has greatly declined, arsenic is still used as a pesticide, particularly in growing cotton, as a herbicide, and as a wood preservative.

Arsenic poisoning from well water remains a serious worldwide human health concern. Internationally, in West Bengal and Bangladesh more than 75 million people are exposed to arsenic-laden water that threatens their health. People of Argentina, Chile, and Taiwan also have elevated arsenic in their drinking water. In the United States, federal agencies fiercely debate arsenic drinking-water standards, which would limit the amount of arsenic in municipal wells. This is particularly relevant to areas of western United States that have elevated arsenic in their drinking water.

Arsenic is a versatile metal, forming various compounds, either inorganic or organic, with a complex chemistry. Inorganic arsenic is widely distributed in nature, usually in the trivalent form ($As^{3+}$) but also as pentavalent arsenic ($As^{5+}$). The trivalent forms include arsenic trioxide, sodium arsenite, and arsenic trichloride. Organic arsenic, much less toxic than inorganic arsenic, is produced in a biomethylation process by many organisms including humans and shellfish.

Arsenic use and production has declined with recognition of its toxicity and the development of suitable replacements. It is not mined but produced as a byproduct of smelting for copper, lead, and zinc. The last US smelter producing arsenic in Tacoma, Washington closed in 1985. Smelters typically released the trivalent arsenic trioxide and lead into the atmosphere, which contaminated the local environment leaving an unwelcome legacy for local residents. Approximately 20,000 tons of arsenic are imported into the United States with about 90% of that being used as a wood preservative in lumber pressure-treated with chromate, copper, and arsenate. This use of arsenic is also being phased out to some degree. Arsenic is used in the manufacture of silicon-based computer chip technology and in glass manufacture to control color. Inorganic arsenic is no longer used as a pesticide in cotton fields and orchards, but some forms of organic arsenic continue to be applied to cotton fields. Inorganic arsenic is also released from coal-fired electric generation facilities, and cigarette smokers inhale some arsenic from tobacco. Organic arsenic compounds are also used as a feed additive to enhance growth of poultry and swine.

We are exposed to constant but low levels of arsenic, unless exposed in an occupational setting or to arsenic-contaminated drinking water. Normally the background air contains less than 0.1 $\mu g/m^3$ and drinking water less than 5 $\mu g/l$, but water levels can be significantly higher. Food usually supplies less than 10 $\mu g/day$ of arsenic but can be higher with the consumption of fish and particularly shellfish, which can have arsenic levels up to 30 $\mu g/g$. The majority of arsenic in food is inorganic with a low level of toxicity. The total average daily exposure to arsenic is about 20 $\mu g/day$ from food and water (assume 2000 ml/day average water consumption at 5 $\mu g/l$ arsenic). Children have higher levels of exposure, particularly if drinking water concentrations of arsenic are elevated, because of their smaller size and greater consumption of water relative to their size. Several state health departments and public interest groups have expressed concern about children repeatedly exposed to arsenic from playing on arsenic-treated deck or play structures. Some exposure and associated risk calculations exceed the EPA's acceptable risk levels. Arsenic exposure can also occur if arsenic-treated wood is burned or from breathing sawdust from treated wood.

## 9.4 Biological properties

Soluble inorganic arsenic compounds, such as arsenic trioxide, are readily absorbed from the intestine (80–90%). Organic arsenic compounds found in seafood are not well absorbed. Arsenic can also be absorbed through the lungs and skin. Most of the arsenic in the blood is bound to red blood cells. Once ingested, inorganic arsenic is biotransformed by the liver to a methylated form of arsenic and excreted in the urine with a half-life of 3 to 5 days. Arsenic is also excreted in the outer layer of skin cells and sweat. Arsenic binds to sulfhydryl-containing proteins and concentrates in the hair and fingernails. At higher levels of exposure, white bands, called Mees' lines, are visible in the nails.

## 9.5 Health effects

They put arsenic in his meat
And stared aghast to watch him eat;
They poured strychnine in his cup
And shook to see him drink it up
　A. E. (Alfred Edward) Housman (1859–1936).

The acute effects of inorganic arsenic poisoning are well known from the incidence of suicidal, homicidal, and accidental poisonings. Ingestion of 70 to 180 mg of arsenic trioxide can be fatal, but initial effects may be delayed for several hours. Symptoms following oral ingestion include constriction of the throat with difficulty in swallowing, severe intestinal pain, vomiting, diarrhea, muscle cramps, severe thirst, coma, and death. If the patient survives the acute symptoms, there is often peripheral nervous system damage.

The symptoms of chronic arsenic exposure are most often associated with contaminated drinking water. Early signs of arsenic exposure are garlic odor on the breath, excessive perspiration, muscle tenderness and weakness, and changes in skin pigmentation. More advanced symptoms include anemia, reduced sensation in the hands and feet from damage to the peripheral sensory system (stocking and glove syndrome), peripheral vascular disease, skin changes on palms and soles, and liver and kidney involvement. Changes in circulation can lead to gangrene of extremities, especially of the feet, which has been referred to as Blackfoot disease. Hyperpigmentation and hyperkeratosis of palms and soles occurs in 3 to 6 months with repeated ingestion of 0.4 mg/kg per day. Many of the symptoms are dose and time dependent. In other words, repeated low levels of exposure over an extended period of time can produce similar effects to a one-time high level of exposure.

Arsenic causes both skin and lung cancer. Skin cancer was observed over 100 years ago in patients treated with arsenical compounds, and lung cancer was seen in smelter workers who chronically inhaled arsenic dust. Although arsenic is an established human carcinogen, it has been difficult to confirm and study in animal models. Arsenic readily crosses the placenta, but there appears to be increased methylation of arsenic to its organic form, which reduces its toxicity to the fetus.

## 9.6 Reducing exposure

The only supernatural agents, which can in any manner be allowed to us moderns, are ghosts; but of these I would advise an author to be extremely sparing. These are indeed, like arsenic, and other dangerous drugs in physic, to be used with the utmost caution . . .

Henry Fielding, 1917.

The toxicity of chronic exposure to arsenic is well established and the best recommendation is to avoid arsenic exposure. The most common home exposure is from contaminated drinking water and arsenic-treated lumber. Certain areas of the country have higher levels of arsenic in water. The EPA has lowered arsenic drinking water standards, but water providers have until 2006 to meet the new standards. Avoid inhalation of sawdust from arsenic-treated lumber or inhalation of smoke from burning arsenic-treated wood. And of course always wash your hands. This is particularly important if a young child is playing on arsenic-treated wood.

Families with decks, play equipment, furniture, or other structures made with arsenic-treated lumber should take steps to reduce exposure, especially to children. Home uses of arsenic-treated lumber are being phased out in the United States, but it is estimated that approximately 60 billion board feet of arsenic-treated lumber is still in use in the United States as of 2002, about enough to cover half the state of California with a deck two inches thick. Several state agencies have recommended that treated lumber on which children may play should be coated periodically with paint or other sealer to reduce hand contact and subsequent ingestion of arsenic. Those who choose to remove arsenic-treated decks or other structures may want to test the soil underneath to see if levels exceed state standards.

## 9.7 Regulatory standards

- EPA – Drinking water 10 µg/l (10 ppb)
- EPA – RfD – 0.3 µg/kg per day (chronic exposure)
- OSHA – Workplace air – 0.5 mg/m$^3$
- ATSDR – MRL – 0.3 µg/kg per day (chronic exposure)

## 9.8 Recommendation and conclusions

Arsenic is an ancient and well-known hazard and, along with lead and mercury, is an important environmental contaminant. The inorganic form is far more toxic than organic arsenic, which is commonly found in seafood. Arsenic-contaminated drinking water is a worldwide problem that affects millions of people. Human exposure also occurs from arsenic-treated lumber.

The best recommendation is to avoid or reduce exposure to inorganic arsenic.

## 9.9 More information and references

### 9.9.1 Slide presentation

- A Small Dose of Arsenic presentation material. Online. Available HTTP: <http://www.crcpress.com/e_products/> and follow the links to downloads and then the catalog number TF1691.
  Web site contains presentation material related to the health effects of arsenic.

### 9.9.2 European, Asian, and international agencies

- World Health Organization (WHO). Online. Available HTTP: <http://www.who.int/inf-fs/en/fact210.html> (accessed: 9 April 2003).
  Arsenic fact sheet.

### 9.9.3 North American agencies

- Health Canada – Arsenic in Drinking Water. Online. Available HTTP: <http://www.hc-sc.gc.ca/english/iyh/environment/arsenic.html> (accessed: 9 April 2003).
  Health Canada provides information on the health effects of arsenic in drinking water.
- US Food and Drug Administration (FDA). Online. Available HTTP: <http://www.cfsan.fda.gov/~frf/guid-as.html> (accessed: 9 April 2003).
  FDA Guidance Document for Arsenic in Shellfish.
- US Environmental Protection Agency (EPA). Online. Available HTTP: <http://www.epa.gov/> (accessed: 9 April 2003).
  Site has general information and research on arsenic.
- US Environmental Protection Agency (EPA) – Integrated Risk Information System. Online. Available HTTP: <http://www.epa.gov/iriswebp/iris/> (accessed: 9 April 2003).
  Site contains EPA's risk assessment evaluation of arsenic.
- US Environmental Protection Agency (EPA) – Toxics Release Inventory (TRI) Program. Online. Available HTTP: <http://www.epa.gov/tri/> (accessed: 9 April 2003).
  Site has information on arsenic release in the United States.
- US ATSDR – Agency for Toxic Substance Disease Registry – Toxicology Profile Series Arsenic. Online. Available HTTP: <http://www.atsdr.cdc.gov/ToxProfiles/> (accessed: 9 April 2003).
- US National Research Council (NRC) – Arsenic in Drinking Water: 2001 Update. Online. Available HTTP: <http://www.nationalacademies.org/publications/> (accessed: 9 April 2003).
  The NRC report on arsenic can be accessed from their web site.
- US Geological Services (USGS). Online. Available HTTP: <http://co.water.usgs.gov/trace/arsenic/> (accessed: 9 April 2003).
  Site contains a map of the United States showing arsenic in water.

## 9.9.4 Non-government organizations

- Arsenic Crisis Information Center – Arsenic in West Bengal & Bangladesh. Online. Available HTTP: <http://bicn.com/acic/> (accessed: 9 April 2003). Site has information and pictures related to arsenic poisoning in West Bengal and Bangladesh.
- Harvard University. Online. Available HTTP: <http://phys4.harvard.edu/~wilson/arsenic_project_main.html> (accessed: 9 April 2003). Site has information on health effects of chronic arsenic poisoning.

## 9.9.5 References

- Environmentally healthy homes and communities. Children's special vulnerabilities. (2001). Am Nurse, 33(6), 26–38; quiz 39–40.
- Hall, A. H. (2002). Chronic arsenic poisoning. Toxicol Lett, 128(1–3), 69–72.
- Jiang, J. Q. (2001). Removing arsenic from groundwater for the developing world – a review. Water Sci Technol, 44(6), 89–98.
- Liu, J., Zheng, B., Aposhian, H. V., Zhou, Y., Chen, M. L., Zhang, A. and Waalkes, M. P. (2002). Chronic arsenic poisoning from burning high-arsenic-containing coal in Guizhou, China. Environ Health Perspect, 110(2), 119–122.
- Pott, W. A., Benjamin, S. A. and Yang, R. S. (2001). Pharmacokinetics, metabolism, and carcinogenicity of arsenic. Rev Environ Contam Toxicol, 169, 165–214.
- Rahman, M. M., Chowdhury, U. K., Mukherjee, S. C., Mondal, B. K., Paul, K., Lodh, D., Biswas, B. K., Chanda, C. R., Basu, G. K., Saha, K. C., Roy, S., Das, R., Palit, S. K., Quamruzzaman, Q. and Chakraborti, D. (2001). Chronic arsenic toxicity in Bangladesh and West Bengal, India – a review and commentary. J Toxicol Clin Toxicol, 39(7), 683–700.
- Smith, A. H., Lingas, E. O. and Rahman, M. (2000). Contamination of drinking-water by arsenic in Bangladesh: a public health emergency. Bull World Health Org, 78(9), 1093–1103.
- WHO. (2000). Towards an Assessment of Socioeconomic Impact of Arsenic Poisoning in Bangladesh. World Health Organization, Sustainable Development and Healthy Environments, WHO/SDE/WSH/00.4, 1–42.
- Yu, H. S., Lee, C. H., Jee, S. H., Ho, C. K. and Guo, Y. L. (2001). Environmental and occupational skin diseases in Taiwan. J Dermatol, 28(11), 628–631.

# Chapter 10

## Metals

## Contents

- Introduction
- Nutritionally important metals
- Toxicologically important metals
- Medically important metals
- Chelating agents
- Fluoride
- More information and references

## 10.1 Introduction

Metals are essential for humans and indeed for all life. We began using metals to build and shape our society over 4000 years ago. The Greeks and Romans were some of the first to document both the toxic and potential healing effects of metals. Arsenic was well known both as a poison and treatment for disease.

The use of metals in our industrialized society has significantly altered the natural distribution of metals in the environment. Our progress and folly is well documented in the Greenland ice. Lead in the Greenland ice began increasing about 800 BC, documenting its use and redistribution as civilizations flourished and declined. A dramatic increase occurred when lead was added to gasoline in the 1920s. Overall there has been a 200-fold increase in lead in the Greenland ice due to human use of lead.

Metals cannot be created or destroyed, but can change form, altering their biological availability and toxicity. Metallic mercury evaporates and is redistributed from the atmosphere across the globe. When the mercury is retuned to land or water, bacteria form methyl mercury ($Hg$-$CH_3$), which is then taken up by increasingly larger organisms and ultimately ends up in fish, such as tuna, that humans and other animals consume.

The principles of toxicology, dose – response and individual sensitivity, are well illustrated by the metals. Historically, most of the interest and concern was with the obvious effects of metal toxicity such as colic from lead or symptoms of the "Mad Hatter" from mercury. The emphasis has changed to the more subtle and long-term effects and concern for potentially sensitive individuals. It is now well documented that children exposed to even low levels of lead will have a lowered IQ and other learning difficulties. This knowledge has resulted in significant changes in our use of metals.

In this chapter, the metals are divided into three sections:

(1) nutritionally important metals or essential metals
(2) important toxic metals
(3) medically useful metals.

There is also a very brief section on chelating agents used to treat over-exposure to metals Finally, fluoride is mentioned as a medically important compound. Only selected metals are reviewed and the reviews are very brief, covering key points about their biological activity and toxic effects. The accompanying presentation material has one slide for each metal highlighting key facts. Three metals, arsenic, lead, and mercury, are covered in more detail in separate chapters. These three metals are recognized as persistent environmental contaminants and are toxicologically important.

## 10.2 Nutritionally important metals

### 10.2.1 Introduction

Our very existence is dependent on a number of metals, the most common of which is iron. Some of the more important ones are described below. As essential elements, the beneficial and adverse effects of these metals have been carefully studied and recommendations developed on daily intake. These recommendations are generally very broad and can vary depending on age – child or adult, young or old – or during pregnancy. The recommended daily intakes quoted below are for adults. These recommendations are actually oral exposure levels with intestinal absorption highly variable and dependent on the metal and other variables. A quick look at a typical cereal box will demonstrate the importance placed on these elements.

Since they are essential for life, the toxicity of these metals can result from either nutritional deficiency or excess exposure, but the focus will be on excess exposure. However, nutritional iron deficiency is worth mentioning, as it is a problem in the United States as well as worldwide and lack of iron can contribute to lead toxicity. Depending on the route of exposure, metal toxicity can be very different. Metals like zinc and manganese can be very toxic when inhaled. As we have seen with many agents, there is a beneficial and a hazardous side depending on route of

**Table 10.1 Summary of nutritionally important metals**

| Metal | Function | Source | Toxicity (when in excess) | Recommended daily allowance |
|---|---|---|---|---|
| Chromium (Cr) | Associated with insulin | Food supply | Kidney damage, lung cancer (inhalation) | 50 to 200 µg ($Cr^{3+}$) |
| Copper (Cu) | Synthesis of hemoglobin | Food supply | Toxicity is very rare, deficiency – anemia; excess – liver and kidney | 1.5 to 3.0 mg |
| Iron (Fe) | Hemoglobin | Food supply | Intestinal tract, liver damage | 10 to 15 mg |
| Magnesium (Mg) | Associated with many enzymes | Food supply | Inhalation in welding | 280 to 350 mg |
| Manganese (Mn) | Associated with many enzymes | Food supply, grains and nuts | Parkinson's-like syndrome | 2 to 5 mg |
| Selenium (Se) | Anticancer | Food supply | Heart | 55 to 70 µg |
| Zinc (Zn) | Associated with many enzymes | Food supply | Deficiency – impaired growth | 12 to 15 mg |

exposure and amount of exposure. The nutritionally important metals are summarized in Table 10.1.

## 10.2.2 Chromium (Cr)

Chromium is an abundant and essential element that exists in oxidation states from $Cr^{2+}$ to $Cr^{6+}$, of which $Cr^{3+}$ is biologically important and $Cr^{6+}$ industrially important. $Cr^{3+}$ is associated with insulin and regulation of glucose. Recommended daily intake is 50 to 200 µg. Chromium ($Cr^{6+}$) has a range of industrial uses including as an alloy in stainless steel and in tanning leather. The most serious industrial exposure is by inhalation and is most prominent in chrome production and plating industries. Acute chromium exposure causes kidney damage and skin contact can cause contact dermatitis and when inhaled irritate the nasal lining. It should also be considered a lung carcinogen.

## 10.2.3 Copper (Cu)

Copper is involved in hemoglobin synthesis and toxicity is rare either from deficiency or excess. Recommended daily intake is 1.5 to 3.0 mg. It is widely used in a number of products including plumbing and electrical wire and is readily available in the food supply. Copper deficiency has been associated with anemia but is generally associated with broader nutritional problems. Grazing animals, for example cattle, can ingest too much copper, affecting the liver and kidney. In humans, Wilson's disease, a genetic inability to metabolize copper, can be treated with the chelator penicillamine.

### 10.2.4 Iron (Fe)

There is 3 to 5 grams of iron in the body and two-thirds of that is associated with the oxygen-carrying hemoglobin of the red blood cells. Recommended daily intake is 10 to 15 mg, but this increases to 30 mg during pregnancy. Iron deficiency is the most common nutritional deficiency worldwide, affecting children and adults. Iron deficiency results in anemia or a decrease in the oxygen-carrying capacity of the blood. The intestinal tract actively transports iron and, if there is low iron in the diet, other metals such as lead will be absorbed, resulting in increased lead toxicity. Before the introduction of child-proof caps for medicine, children were often treated for the acute effects of iron toxicity after ingesting iron supplements, suffering vomiting, liver damage, shock, kidney failure, and possibly death. Chronic excess exposure to iron can result in ulceration of the intestinal tract, which in turn results in bloody vomit and black feces.

### 10.2.5 Magnesium (Mg)

Magnesium, a nutritionally essential metal, is found in grains, seafood, nuts, meats, and drinking water. Recommended daily intake ranges from 280 to 350 mg per day for adult females and males, respectively. It is also used in a number of antacids and cathartics. Milk of magnesia or magnesium hydroxide is known as a universal antidote for poisoning. Magnesium is a cofactor in a number of essential enzymes and involved in several key metabolic reactions. Magnesium is primarily absorbed in the small intestine and is routinely excreted in the urine at about 12 mg/day. Magnesium blood levels are constant and consistently regulated.

Magnesium deficiency, usually the result of decreased absorption or excessive excretion, results in neuromuscular weakness and ultimately convulsions. Dietary deficiency in cattle is known as the grass staggers. Magnesium toxicity from impaired excretion or excessive consumption of antacids results in vomiting, hypertension, and central nervous systems effects. Inhalation of magnesium oxide from welding can cause metal fume fever similar to that from zinc.

### 10.2.6 Manganese (Mn)

Manganese is an essential element involved in numerous enzymatic reactions, particularly those associated with the fatty acids. Intestinal tract absorption is poor (less that 5%) but it is readily available in foods such as grains, fruits, nuts, and tea. Recommended daily intake is 2 to 5 mg. There is increased interest in the toxicity of manganese because of its use in the gasoline additive, as MMT (methylcyclopentadienyl Mn tricarbonyl), which results in manganese salts being distributed into the environment from the tail pipes of cars. Manganese is also an important alloy in steel. Inhalation exposure during mining or steel production can cause respiratory disease. Manganese exposure can also result in a serious nervous system disease that resembles the movement disorders of Parkinson's disease, characterized by difficulty walking, irritability, and speech difficulties. There is ongoing research on the potential adverse effects from use as a fuel additive.

### 10.2.7 Selenium (Se)

Selenium is readily available in a variety of foods including shrimp, meat, dairy products, and grains, with a recommended daily intake of 55 to 70 μg. It occurs in several forms with $Se^{+6}$ being biologically most important. Selenium is readily absorbed by the intestine and is widely distributed throughout the tissues of the body, with the highest levels in the liver and kidney. It is active in a variety of cellular functions and interacts with vitamin E. Selenium appears to reduce the toxic effects of metals such as cadmium and mercury and to have anticarcinogenic activity. Selenium produces notable adverse effects both in deficiency and excess; thus recommended daily intake for adults is approximately 70 μg/day but should not exceed 200 μg/day.

Excess selenium intake can occur in both animals and humans living in areas with elevated selenium in the soil. Most grass and grains do not accumulate selenium, but when an animal consumes plants that do accumulate selenium (some up to 10,000 mg/kg) they can develop a condition called the "blind staggers". Symptoms include depressed appetite, impaired vision, and staggering in circles and can ultimately lead to paralysis and death. Humans are susceptible to similar effects as well as additional neurological effects. Selenium deficiency results in heart disorders, skeletal muscle effects, and liver damage.

### 10.2.8 Zinc (Zn)

Zinc plays a number of important roles in the body and deficiency results in serious adverse effects. Recommended daily intake is 12 to 15 mg. Zinc is very common in the environment and readily available in many foods, including grains, nuts, legumes, meats, seafood, and dairy products. Numerous enzymes require zinc, as do proteins that regulate gene expression. Zinc plays a role in the immune system and is also important in the development and function of the nervous system.

Zinc deficiency during fetal or infant development can lead to impaired growth, increased illness, impaired healing, loss of hair, and central nervous system disorders. Some studies have linked adult zinc deficiency with neurological disorders such as Alzheimer's disease. Diseases associated with zinc deficiency are linked to liver disorders from alcoholism. A number of drugs, particularly chelating agents and some antibiotics, affect zinc homeostasis. Exposure to zinc and other metals during welding can cause metal fume fever, characterized by chills, fever, weakness, and sweating.

## 10.3 Toxicologically important metals

### 10.3.1 Introduction

While some metals are nutritionally important, there is another group with no beneficial biological effects and in some cases serious toxic effects. Our complex relationship with metals is well illustrated by lead, which we have used for a variety of purposes since ancient times. In the last hundred years, lead was extensively used in paint and as a gasoline fuel additive. In the last 30 years, it was recognized

**Table 10.2 Summary of toxic metals**

| Metal | Toxic effects | Source |
|---|---|---|
| Aluminum (Al) | Dialysis dementia | During dialysis, food, drinking water, |
| Arsenic (As) (can exist in different forms) | Cancer (skin and lung) Neurotoxic (sensory effects) Liver and vascular | Drinking water, smelting of ore, used in pesticides, treated wood |
| Beryllium (Be) | Lung, hypersensitivity, delayed and progressive effects (berylliosis), contact dermatitis | Nuclear power plants, alloy in metals, coal combustion |
| Cadmium (Cd) | Lung, emphysema, kidney, calcium metabolism, possible lung carcinogen | Shellfish, cigarette smoke, taken up by plants, metal alloy – welding |
| Cobalt (Co) | Inhalation exposure "hard metal" pneumoconiosis | Alloy in metals – but also associated with vitamin $B_{12}$ |
| Lead (Pb) | Decreased learning and memory (children very sensitive) | Old paint, food, formerly used as a gasoline additive |
| Mercury – inorganic (Hg) | Tremor, excitability, memory lose, the "Mad Hatter" | Thermometers, switches, fluorescent lights |
| Mercury – organic (Hg-$CH_3$) | Tremor, developmental effects on nervous system | Fish |
| Nickel (Ni) | Lung carcinogen, contact dermatitis | Food supply, workplace exposure |
| Tin (Sn) | Inorganic – low, lung Organic – central nervous system | Inorganic – food packaging, dust; organic – rare |

that children exposed to even low levels of lead could suffer permanent brain damage and reduced intelligence. This worldwide use and distribution of lead has had significant effects on individuals as well as society as a whole. There is a somewhat similar story for mercury. The examples of lead and mercury clearly illustrate the fundamental principles of toxicology – dose–response and individual sensitivity. The toxic metals are summarized in Table 10.2.

## 10.3.2 Aluminum (Al)

Aluminum was first isolated in 1825 and is now recognized as the most abundant metal in the environment. Historically, this abundance has not translated into biological availability because it is highly reactive and remains bound to a range of elements. However, acid rain has increased the bioavailability of aluminum in the environment. Aluminum is used in a wide range of products from airplanes, to beer and soft drink cans, to cooking pans. Human exposure to aluminum is from drinking water, food, and some drugs. Daily intake ranges from 1 to 10 mg, but it is poorly absorbed in the intestine. Aluminum does not appear to have any essential biological function.

The neurotoxic effects of aluminum were first observed in people undergoing dialysis for treatment of kidney failure. This syndrome, called dialysis dementia, starts with speech disorders and progresses to dementia and convulsions. Symptoms corresponded with elevated aluminum levels commonly found in bone, brain, and muscle following 3 to 7 years of treatment. Elevated levels of aluminum were also found in the brains of people suffering from Alzheimer's disease. Despite considerable research, it is not clear if the aluminum accumulation in the brain is a cause of Alzheimer's disease or a result of changes in the brain associated with the disease.

### 10.3.3 Arsenic (As)

Arsenic has a colorful history, having been used with great effect as a poison and also to treat a variety of ailments, including cancer. Its properties were first studied over 2000 years ago and contributed to some of the first theories on toxicology. Despite its toxicity, arsenic was still found in cosmetics into the twentieth century. Prior to the recognition of the toxic properties of arsenic, it was widely used as a pesticide in orchards, which resulted in soil contamination. The vast majority of treated wood in residential decks and other structures contains arsenic. Workplace exposure occurs in the smelting of ore, and arsenic is also widely used in the electronic manufacturing industry. Of considerable public concern, which has resulted in several large studies by the government, is the presence of arsenic in drinking water. Some municipal or well waters can contain elevated arsenic levels.

Chemically, arsenic is complex in that it can exist in a variety of forms including trivalent and pentavalent or as arsenic trioxide (computer chip manufacture) and arsenic acid. Arsenic is excreted in skin cells, sweat, hair, and fingernails, which can be seen as white transverse bands. Acute exposure to arsenic results in gastrointestinal pain, sensory loss, cardiovascular failure, and death. Chronic exposure or survival of acute exposure can cause loss of peripheral sensory function and loss of central nervous system function. Chronic arsenic exposure can also cause cancer of the lung and skin (see the chapter on arsenic).

### 10.3.4 Beryllium (Be)

Beryllium is an important metal alloy used in the nuclear power industry. Its presence in coal and oil results in more than 1250 tons being released into the environment annually from fuel combustion at power plants. Exposure is primarily from inhalation, but skin contact can result in dermatitis. Cigarette smokers also inhale a little beryllium. Initially, beryllium distributes to the liver, but ultimately is absorbed by bone.

Contact dermatitis and hypersensitivity to beryllium is the most common toxic reaction. Workplace inhalation of beryllium can be very serious. Acute exposure can result in an inflammatory reaction along the entire respiratory tract. Chronic beryllium disease or berylliosis can result from chronic workplace exposure. This is a serious and progressive degenerative disease in which the lungs become increasingly fibrotic and dysfunctional. Long-term exposure can result in lung cancer, and beryllium is classified as a carcinogen by international regulatory agencies.

### *10.3.5 Cadmium (Cd)*

Cadmium is a widely distributed metal used in manufacturing and is present in a number of consumer products. Dietary exposure to cadmium is possible from shellfish and plants grown on cadmium-contaminated soils. Absorption is increased when associated with low levels of iron or calcium in the diet. Some plants, such as tobacco, can concentrate cadmium from even low levels in the soil. The lung readily absorbs cadmium, thus cigarette smokers have elevated cadmium exposure. Cadmium is also used as a metal alloy, in paint, and in batteries (Ni-Cad, nickel–cadmium). Workplace exposure can occur in welding and battery manufacture.

Oral ingestion of cadmium results in less than 10% absorption, but inhalation exposure results in much higher absorption through the lungs. Cadmium accumulates in the liver and kidney, with the kidney being particularly important in binding cadmium and reducing its toxicity. Ingestion of high levels from acute exposure can result in abdominal pain, nausea, and vomiting while inhalation exposure results in impaired breathing (pulmonary edema or accumulation of fluid in the lungs). Chronic exposure can result in obstructive lung disease, emphysema, and kidney disease. Cadmium may also be related to increases in blood pressure (hypertension) and is a possible lung carcinogen. Cadmium affects calcium metabolism and can result in bone loss. This condition has been referred to as "Itai-Itai" disease, which means "Ouch-Ouch" in Japanese and reflects the bone pain associated with cadmium effects on calcium.

### *10.3.6 Cobalt (Co)*

Cobalt in small amounts is an essential element associated with vitamin $B_{12}$, but at high levels can be toxic. There are no daily recommended intake levels for cobalt. Intestinal bacteria use cobalt to produce cobalamin, which in turn is an essential component of vitamin $B_{12}$. Industrially, cobalt is used in pigments, permanent magnets, and as an alloy to harden metals as in tungsten carbide blades or drills.

High chronic oral consumption of cobalt has been used to treat anemia but can also cause goiter. High acute consumption of cobalt can cause vomiting, diarrhea, a sensation of warmth, and heart failure. The last was noted during a period when cobalt was added to beer to improve foaming. When inhaled, for example in metal grinding for sharpening, cobalt can cause "hard metal" pneumoconiosis, a progressive disease of the lungs.

### *10.3.7 Lead (Pb)*

Lead was as important in the Roman Empire as it was in the twentieth century and its use almost equally as disastrous. In the Roman Empire, lead's malleability and low melting point made it ideal for plumbing, not unlike its use in solder in plumbing, centuries later, that can be found in many households. The Romans also added lead to wine as a sweetener and preservative. In the twentieth century, lead was commonly added to paint, sometimes as much as 50%, which in fact created an excellent, long-lasting paint. But the sweetness of lead attracted children who readily consumed lead paint chips, a behavior referred to as pica. Due to its low melting point, lead was used as solder in tin cans containing food and in plumbing. In what some refer to as the greatest public health disaster of the twentieth century, lead was added to gasoline to improve car engine durability. Lead was emitted from the tail pipes of cars, contaminating both local and distant areas. Children absorb up to 50% of lead that is orally ingested, as it substitutes for the much needed calcium. This is in contrast to adults, who only absorb about 10% of orally ingested lead. Lead is still a serious concern in areas near smelters and housing with lead-based paint. As the toxicity of lead at lower levels was recognized it was banned from paint and from gasoline.

The Greek Dioscorides recognized the health effects of lead in the 2nd century BC when he stated, "Lead makes the mind give way". In the 1700s Benjamin Franklin noted that lead exposure caused the "dry gripes", or stomach upset. Painters that used lead-based paint suffered from "wrist drop" caused by the effects of lead on the peripheral nervous system. At the turn of the twentieth century it was recognized that children seemed to be particularly sensitive to high levels of lead that resulted in swelling of the brain, kidney disease, effects on hemoglobin, and possible death. In the 1970s, studies demonstrated that even low levels of lead exposure harmed the developing nervous system. It is now well accepted that lead is a very potent neurotoxicant. Australia banned the use of lead in paint in the 1920s, but this step was not taken until 50 years later in the US. On average, the biggest drop in the blood lead levels of children occurred following the phase out of lead in gasoline in the 1980s. The US Centers for Disease Prevention and Control (CDC) have established a blood lead level of 10 µg/dl or greater as an action level. There is no safety factor associated with this level and there is sufficient data to indicate that the nervous system of children is damaged at blood lead levels of 10 µg/dl (see chapter on lead).

### 10.3.8 Mercury – inorganic (Hg)

Inorganic mercury is a silvery colored liquid at room temperature. Many people have had the opportunity to "play" with mercury, coating pennies and pushing it around on a flat surface. Now we know that the mercury was evaporating and that there are serious health consequences to the inhalation of mercury vapor. Due to its reactive properties and ability to combine with other metals, inorganic mercury is used at nuclear weapon facilities and in gold mining. In the gold mining process, the ore is mixed with mercury and the metallic mixture heated to evaporate the mercury leaving the gold behind. This process results in a significant release of mercury into the atmosphere. The atmospheric circulation of mercury has made it an important worldwide contaminant. When returned to the earth or water, inorganic mercury is converted into an organic mercury compound (see below). Although there are growing efforts to phase out the use of mercury from consumer products, it has been widely distributed in thermometers, switches (thermostats and car boot lid switches), fluorescent light bulbs, and scientific instruments such as those used in measuring blood pressure. Many of us have mercury in our mouths as a dental amalgam with silver. Dental fillings contain approximately 50% mercury. This use of mercury has resulted in crematoria being an important source of atmospheric release. Dental surgeries are also an important source of mercury entering the waste stream and then into the environment. Mercury has also been used to treat a variety of diseases including syphilis. Coal contains mercury, and combustion of coal at power plants is a significant source of atmospheric mercury. While human activity has greatly contributed to the release of mercury, some release occurs naturally from soil containing mercury and volcanic activity.

The toxic effects of mercury vapor have been well documented and even recorded in the literature as the "Mad Hatter" in Lewis Carroll's *Alice in Wonderland*. Mercury was used to cure the felt used in hats, and workers developed the characteristic signs of mercury vapor toxicity. Acute exposure to high concentrations of mercury vapor causes respiratory distress, which can be fatal. The symptoms of chronic exposure to mercury vapor include personality changes such as excitability, depression, memory loss, fine motor tremor that can become progressively worse, gingivitis, and hallucination. There is some mercury inhalation exposure from dental amalgam, but for most people there are no health-related effects. Metallic mercury is very poorly absorbed from the intestine, thus it is much better to swallow the mercury from a thermometer than inhale it (see chapter on mercury).

### 10.3.9 Mercury – organic (Hg-CH$_3$)

There are several different types of organic mercury, but by far the most important in terms of health effects is methyl mercury. When atmospheric mercury is deposited on the ground or in the water, it is converted to methyl mercury by bacteria. Mercury compounds are very toxic and this is the bacteria's way to detoxify mercury. Small animals then consume the bacteria, along with the methyl mercury and bigger animals in turn consume the smaller animals, thus increasing the concentrations of methyl mercury. Methyl mercury accumulates in the larger carnivorous animals, most important of which are fish such as tuna, pike, and shark. Mercury accumulates in the muscle of the fish, which makes it all but impossible to avoid consumption of the methyl mercury. Methyl mercury is readily absorbed from the intestine and crosses the blood–brain barrier and the placenta.

The devastating health effects were first documented in Minamata, Japan in the late 1950s chiefly among fishermen and their families. A subsequent mercury-poisoning incident took place in Iraq when people consumed seed grain coated with organic mercury fungicides. Both of these incidents, as well as others, affected thousands of people and clearly demonstrated the most significant adverse developmental effects of mercury exposure. Early stage effects include tingling and numbness around the mouth and lips and may extend to the fingers and toes. Continued exposure can result in difficulty walking, fatigue, inability to concentrate, loss of vision, tremor, and eventually death. The developing fetus and young children are particularly sensitive to the effects of methyl mercury exposure. The serious health effects of mercury combined with its widespread distribution have resulted in numerous health advisories and restriction on fish consumption. Typically, children and women of childbearing age are advised to limit their consumption of species of fish known to accumulate mercury. The US Food and Drug Administration limits the amount of mercury in canned tuna to 1 ppm (see chapter on mercury).

### 10.3.10 Nickel (Ni)

Nickel is widely used as a metal alloy in stainless steel, where it increases hardness and corrosion resistance. It is generally present in the environment and appears to be an essential element for some plant life and bacteria. It is available in low concentrations in the food supply. The most serious workplace exposure is from inhalation. Exposure to the general population is from jewelry, cooking utensils, and other metals containing nickel. For the general population, the primary health concern is an allergic response from skin contact. In the workplace, inhalation of nickel compounds can cause respiratory tract cancer, particularly lung and nasal cancers. Nickel is one of the few proven human carcinogens. Contact dermatitis is also a common workplace hazard.

### 10.3.11 Tin (Sn)

Tin is anther ancient metal that continues to have a variety of uses. The inorganic form is used in food packaging, solder, brass, and as an alloy with other metals. The organic forms of tin, triethyltin and trimethyltin, are used as fungicides, bactericides, and generally as antifouling agents for boats.

Inorganic tin is poorly absorbed in the intestine and toxicity is rare. Prolonged inhalation of tin dust can cause lung disease. Organic tins are readily absorbed by the intestine and are far more toxic. Exposure to organic tins can cause swelling of the brain and cell death in the nervous system.

## 10.4 Medically important metals

### 10.4.1 Introduction

The medical use of metals has declined with the advent of more-targeted drug therapies, but historically metals were used to treat a wide range of human diseases from diarrhea to syphilis and malaria. Currently they are used to treat a limited number of diseases such as ovarian cancer and arthritis, but even this use is in decline. The therapeutic use of metals is generally limited by their toxicity, often causing kidney damage but there can be nervous system damage. Metals are a good example of balancing the benefits of treatment against toxic side effects. The medically important metals are summarized in Table 10.3.

### 10.4.2 Bismuth (Bi)

Bismuth, discovered in 1753, has a long history of medical uses ranging from treatment of syphilis and malaria to diarrhea. More recently, antibacterial properties of bismuth-containing antacids have been used to treat peptic ulcers. In general the medical use of bismuth has declined with the advent of new drug therapies.

Acute toxicity of high-level exposure to bismuth manifests as kidney damage. Chronic low-level exposure to bismuth can result in weakness, joint pain, fever, mental confusion, and difficulty walking. Symptoms usually resolve when exposure is stopped, but can lead to death with ongoing exposure.

### Table 10.3 Summary of medically important metals

| Metal | Function | Source | Toxicity (when in excess) |
|---|---|---|---|
| Bismuth (Bi) | Antacid (ulcers) | Medial, consumer products | Kidney damage |
| Gallium (Ga) | Soft tissue visualization in radiographs | Mining, medical injection | Kidney damage |
| Gold (Au) | Treat rheumatoid arthritis | Mining, medical | Dermatitis, kidney damage |
| Lithium (Li) | Treat psychiatric disorders | Food supply | Tremor, seizures, heart, nausea |
| Platinum (Pt) | Anticancer agent (cisplatin), catalytic converters | Anticancer drug, mining | Kidney, hearing, nervous system |

### 10.4.3 Gallium (Ga)

Gallium, like mercury, is liquid at room temperature, but unlike mercury is much less hazardous. Its most interesting use is as a visualization tool of soft tissues and bone lesions in radiography. Industrial applications include use in high temperature thermometers, metal alloys, and as a substitute for mercury in arc lamps.

Gallium's low toxicity and liquid state at room temperature make it an excellent diagnostic tool. Gallium has a half-life in the body of 4 to 5 days. Higher levels of exposure can cause kidney damage as well as nausea, vomiting, and anemia.

### 10.4.4 Gold (Au)

Gold's aesthetic and electrical properties make it highly desirable and widely used in a number of industrial applications. Medically, gold and gold complexes are used to treat rheumatoid arthritis, but due to its toxicity this use is declining as better treatments become available. Gold has a long half-life in the body.

As with many metals, gold can damage the kidney. Lesions of the mouth and skin are seen following gold therapy to treat arthritis.

### 10.4.5 Lithium (Li)

Lithium was first used to treat manic-depressive illness in 1949, but was not used in the United States until 1970 due to concerns for its toxicity. When used as a therapeutic agent, lithium blood levels must be kept within a very narrow range (i.e., a narrow therapeutic index). Lithium appears to be non-essential, but it is readily absorbed by the intestine and is found in plants and meat. Normal daily intake is about 2 mg. Lithium is used in some manufacturing processes, as a lubricant, and as an alloy.

Outside its therapeutic range, lithium has a wide range of undesirable effects. Nervous system-related effects include tremor, difficulty walking, seizures, slurred speech, and mental confusion. In addition there can be cardiovascular effects, nausea, vomiting, and kidney damage.

### 10.4.6 Platinum (Pt)

Platinum is a relatively rare earth metal usually found with related metals osmium and iridium. While it has a number of industrial applications, its common consumer application is in catalytic converters. This application has actually increased platinum concentrations in roadside dust. The ability of platinum and its derivatives to kill cells or inhibit cell division was discovered in 1965. Platinum-based drugs, such as cisplatin, are used to treat ovarian and testicular cancer, and cancers of the head and neck, as well as others. Unfortunately, the toxic side effects of these agents often limit their usefulness.

In the industrial setting, platinum is relatively harmless, but a few people may be susceptible to developing an allergic skin response (contact dermatitis) and possibly a respiratory response. When used as an anticancer agent, it is typically administered intravenously. It kills cells or inhibits cell division by interfering with DNA synthesis. The most common toxic side effect is kidney damage, but hearing loss, muscular weakness, and peripheral nerve damage are also possible. Platinum is a good example of the benefits and hazards of using a highly toxic drug to treat the uncontrolled cell division of cancer.

## 10.5 Chelating agents

The most obvious treatment of poisoning from excessive metal exposure is to remove the metal from the body, thus the development of chelating agents. While treatment may be necessary, it is far more desirable to prevent exposure. In fact the best treatment for low-level exposure is often to identify the source of exposure and eliminate contact with the metal. An excellent example of this principle is lead, where the most important action is to reduce or eliminate exposure.

While the word chelate comes from the Greek word claw, the development of chelating agents is relatively new. The first chelating agent, BAL (British Anti-Lewisite), was developed during the second World War as a potential treatment for arsenic-based war gases. The ideal chelating agent would bind readily only with the target metal, forming a non-toxic complex that would be excreted easily from the body. Unfortunately, this is easier said than done. BAL, for example, binds with a range of metals, but actually enhances the toxicity of cadmium.

A consistent undesirable property of all chelating agents is that they also complex with essential metals and increase their excretion from the body. The two most common essential metals adversely affected by chelating agents are calcium and zinc. Excessive lead exposure can be treated with the chelating agent calcium-EDTA, not its related sodium salt because this would greatly increase excretion of calcium, potentially having toxic side effects. Blood lead levels are reduced when the lead displaces the calcium to bind with EDTA and is then excreted in the urine. This results in a movement of lead from the soft tissues such as muscle into the blood, which can result in a spike in blood lead levels that may elevate brain lead levels and cause subsequent neurological effects. The lead stored in bone is not affected and will remain until some event mobilizes calcium distribution from the bone. A recent study showed that lead chelation decreased blood lead levels, but did not protect against cognitive deficits.

In summary, while chelating agents can be an effective treatment in some circumstances, they must be approached cautiously. The most important action is to identify the source of exposure and reduce or eliminate it. It is also very important to consider what essential metals may be bound and excreted by the agent. The body tightly regulates most essential metals and disruption of these levels can have serious undesirable (toxic) effects.

## 10.6 Fluoride

Fluoride is widely distributed in soil and is present naturally in drinking water. Fluoride is the salt, such as sodium fluoride, of the element fluorine. It is readily absorbed by the intestine and is incorporated into bone or tooth enamel. When incorporated into teeth, fluoride strengthens the outer layers of enamel, thus reducing dental caries. It is generally accepted that addition of fluoride to the drinking water (approximately 1 ppm) is beneficial for the reduction in childhood dental caries.

Excess exposure to fluoride results in stained or mottled teeth. This is common in areas where fluoride water levels are above 4 ppm. Chronic elevated fluoride exposure can also result in increased bone density. Fluoride has been used to treat decreased bone density.

## 10.7 More information and references

### 10.7.1 Slide presentation

■  A Small Dose of Metals presentation material. Online. Available HTTP: <http://www.crcpress.com/e_products/> and follow the links to downloads and then the catalog number TF1691.
   Web site contains presentation material related to the health effects of many metals.

### 10.7.2 European, Asian, and international agencies

■  England – Department of Health – Nutrition. Online. Available HTTP: <http://www.doh.gov.uk/sacn/index.htm> (accessed: 9 April 2003).
   The Department of Health provides information on nutritional requirements for children and adults.
■  World Health Organization. Online. Available HTTP: <http://www.who.int/en/> (accessed: 4 April 2003).
   Search the health topics section for a specific metal.

### 10.7.3 North American agencies

■ Health Canada – Nutrition. Online. Available HTTP: <http://www.hcsc.gc.ca/english/lifestyles/food_nutr.html> (accessed: 9 April 2003).
Health Canada provides information on nutritional issues.
■ US Agency for Toxic Substance Disease Registry (ATSDR). Online. Available HTTP: <http://www.atsdr.cdc.gov/> (accessed: 4 April 2003).
See fact sheets and case studies on many metals and other agents.

### 10.7.4 Non-government organizations

■ Dartmouth Toxic Metals Research Program. Online. Available HTTP: <http://www.dartmouth.edu/~toxmetal/HM.shtml> (accessed: 4 April 2003).
The site has general information on toxic metals.

### 10.7.5 References

■ Klaassen C. D. (1996). Heavy metals and heavy-metal antagonists. Chapter in Hardman, J. G., Limbird, L. E., Molinoff, P. B., Ruddon, R. W. Gilman, A. G. (eds) *Goodman & Gilman's The Pharmacological Basis of Therapeutics*, 9th edn. McGraw-Hill, New York, pp. 1649–1671.
■ National Academy of Sciences. (1993). Measuring lead exposure in infants, children, and other sensitive populations. National Academy Press: Washington, D.C.
■ Rogan, W. J., Dietrich, K. N., Ware, J. H., Dockery, D. W., Salganik, M., Radcliffe, J., Jones, R. L., Ragan, N. B., Chisolm, J. J., Jr. and Rhoads, G. G. (2001). The effect of chelation therapy with succimer on neuropsychological development in children exposed to lead. N Engl J Med, 344, 1421–1426.

# Chapter 11

# Solvents

## Contents

## 11.1 Dossier

**Name:** solvents (broad class of chemicals)
**Use:** varied – recreational (alcohol) to industrial, gasoline
**Source:** synthetic chemistry, petroleum products, plant oils
**Recommended daily intake:** none (not essential)
**Absorption:** intestine, inhalation (major), skin
**Sensitive individuals:** fetus, children
**Toxicity/symptoms:** nervous system, reproductive system, and death
**General facts:** long history of use (alcohol), high volatility of solvents results in inhalation exposure to vapors
**Environmental:** volatile organic compounds react with sunlight to produce smog
**Recommendations:** avoid, proper workplace protection

## 11.2 Case studies

### 11.2.1 Anesthetic agents

> I also attended on two occasions the operating theatre in the hospital at Edinburgh, and saw two very bad operations, one on a child, but I rushed away before they were completed. Nor did I ever attend again, for hardly any inducement would have been strong enough to make me do so; this being long before the blessed days of chloroform. The two cases fairly haunted me for many a long year.
>
> Charles Darwin (1993).

An effective anesthetic agent must be easy to use, quickly render the patient unconscious, and not produce any toxicity. Dr. William T. G. Morton first publicly demonstrated the use of ether as an effective anesthetic agent at the Massachusetts General Hospital on 16 October 1846 before a crowd of skeptical physicians. Raymundus Lullius, a Spanish chemist, discovered ether $(CH_3CH_2)_2O$ in 1275. Its hypnotic effects were soon appreciated (and enjoyed by some), but for many decades ether was only used to treat the occasional medical ailment. Even with ether, the success of surgical procedures did not improve until the introduction of antiseptic procedures and infection control some 20 years later. Ether was replaced by cyclopropane in 1929, which was replace by halothane in 1956. While anesthetic agents are desirable for the patient, exposure of hospital staff is highly undesirable and an important occupational consideration.

### 11.2.2 n-Hexane

n-Hexane is a simple and common hydrocarbon found in solvents, degreasing agents, glues, spray paints, gasoline, silicones, and other common substances. A common workplace exposure to n-hexane is from degreasing agents, which usually contain a mixture of solvents. In 1997 a 24-year-old male car mechanic went to his doctor complaining of numbness and tingling of the toes and fingers. Further neurological evaluation revealed a reduced sensation in the forearms and diminished reflexes. For the past 22 months this worker used, on a daily basis, aerosol cans of brake cleaner that contained 50–60% hexane (composed of 20%–80% n-hexane), 20–30% toluene, and 1–10% methyl ethyl ketone. He used this degreasing agent to clean brakes, small tools, and even car engines. He commonly used latex gloves while at work. His condition improved when exposure to the cleaning agent was stopped. 2,5-Hexanedione, a urinary metabolite of n-hexane and thought to be the toxic agent responsible for the nervous system effects, can be measured and used to estimate exposure to n-hexane. A subsequent study found that car mechanics were indeed exposed to n-hexane. Degreasing products typically contain a mixture of solvents that are readily absorbed when inhaled or through the skin. The latex gloves used by this worker offered little protection. More information on this case study can be found in MMWR (2001).

## 11.3 Introduction and history

Solvents are a broad class of compounds that we are commonly exposed to when we pump gasoline at the gasoline station, change the car oil, paint the house, glue something back together, drink alcohol, or as an anesthetic when we undergo surgery. Solvents are highly volatile in air and are readily absorbed by the lung when the vapors are inhaled. The small molecular weight of most solvents and their high fat solubility means they are easily absorbed across the skin. Occupational exposure to solvents is common, with an estimated 10 million workers in the United States exposed either though inhalation or skin contact. Acute exposure can result in loss of coordination, reduced speed of response, and general feeling of drunkenness. Long-term exposure can result in decreased learning and memory, reduced ability to concentrate, changes in personality, and even structural changes in the nervous system.

Some people find the effects of solvents on the nervous system desirable and purposely inhale (sniff) solvents to induce a form of intoxication. In the United States approximately 15% of high school students have tried solvent inhalation at least once. Solvents suitable for inhalation and abuse are common in the home. Home products that may contain solvents include paints, paint remover, varnishes, adhesives, glues, degreasing and cleaning agents, dyes, printing ink, floor and shoe polishes, waxes, pesticides, drugs, cosmetics, and fuels, just to name a few (Table 11.1).

In general there are few benefits to solvent exposure and it should be avoided. The one important exception is the use of solvents to induce unconsciousness prior to surgery. As mentioned above, the solvent ether was discovered centuries ago but not used in surgery until the 1840s. Some physicians and dentists first became aware of the effects of ether during "ether frolics" while attending school. Nitrous oxide was also experimented with around the same time, but was not widely adopted by dentists and surgeons until the 1860s. Despite its liver toxicity, chloroform was also used as an anesthetic, particularly in England and Scotland from the late 1840s. Anesthetic agents changed little until the accidental discovery of cyclopropane in 1929. With the increased use of electronic equipment in the surgery area, the flammability of the anesthetic agents became an important issue. In 1956, halothane was discovered by researchers in England, which ushered in a new era in anesthesiology.

**Table 11.1 Products that contain solvents**

| Products that are mostly solvent | Partially solvent based |
| --- | --- |
| Gasoline | Glues |
| Diesel fuel | Adhesives |
| Charcoal lighter fluid | Oil-based paints |
| Lantern fuel | Furniture polishes |
| Grease | Floor polishes and waxes |
| Lubricating oils | Spot removers |
| Degreasing agents | Metal and wood cleaners |
| Paint strippers | Correction fluid |
| Paint thinner | Computer disk cleaner |
| Turpentine | Varnishes and shellacs |
| Nail polish remover | Wood and concrete stains |
| Rubbing alcohol | |

The use of solvents greatly expanded with the industrial revolution, which resulted in widespread release into the environmental. Solvents, such as volatile organic compounds (VOCs), readily evaporate into air, for example when oil-based paint dries. Industrial release also occurs during manufacture or spills. Solvent contamination of drinking water is not uncommon and is a public health issue. VOCs that enter the groundwater become trapped until released during use. Human exposure occurs from drinking water or from exposure during bathing. Solvents such as benzene and trichloroethylene are commonly found at hazardous waste sites.

## 11.4 Biological properties

From a biological perspective the most important properties of solvents are their volatility, high fat solubility (lipophilicity), and small molecule size. Solvents with these characteristics are termed volatile organic compounds. Under normal working conditions solvents readily evaporate into the air, from which they enter the lungs. The high lipid solubility and small size means they are quickly absorbed across lung membranes and enter the blood supply. Blood from the lung moves directly to the brain and other body organs before reaching the liver where metabolism of the solvent occurs. With ongoing exposure, equilibrium is reached between body burden and concentration of the solvent in the air.

Solvents are well absorbed following oral or skin exposure. Most solvents are quickly absorbed from the gut, although the presence of food may delay absorption. Alcohol is a good example of a solvent typically consumed orally. The skin offers little barrier to solvents. Skin exposure to solvents can result in local irritation and increased blood levels of the solvent.

Solvents are eliminated from the body by metabolism or exhalation. The more volatile and fat soluble, the greater the concentration in exhaled air. Exhaled air can be used to estimate solvent concentration in the blood, such as breath analysis for alcohol exposure. Metabolism of solvents occurs primarily in the liver by P450 enzymes. In most cases the metabolism results in reduced toxicity and increased elimination of the resulting products. The toxicity of toluene is reduced when liver enzymes change the compound so that it does not readily cross cell membranes. On the other hand, the toxicity of benzene is increased when it is changed to a compound that can attack the blood-forming cells of the bone marrow causing leukemia. There is considerable variability from one person to the next in their ability to metabolize solvents. Subtle genetic differences can increase or decrease an individual's ability to metabolize certain solvents, resulting in more or less toxicity. The liver is also prone to damage by some solvents, for example carbon tetrachloride ($CCl_4$). This damage can actually be made worse by prior exposure to alcohol.

## 11.5 Health effects

The majority of us are exposed to low levels of solvents every day. Millions of workers around the world are exposed to high levels of solvents on a daily basis that can adversely affect health. Workers often come in contact with more than one solvent during a day's work. Health hazards from solvent exposure range from mild to life threatening, depending on the compound involved and the level and

**Table 11.2 Health effects of solvents**

| Effects of solvents | Examples |
| --- | --- |
| Reproductive hazard | Methoxyethanol, 2-ethoxyethanol, methyl chloride |
| Developmental hazard | Alcohol |
| Liver or kidney damage | Toluene, and carbon tetrachloride, 1,1,2-2-tetrachloroethane, chloroform |
| Nervous system damage | n-Hexane, perchloroethylene, n-butyl mercaptan |
| Cause cancer | Carbon tetrachloride, trichloroethylene, 1,1,2,2-tetrachloroethane, perchloroethylene, methylene chloride, benzene |
| Visual system | Methanol |

duration of exposure. It should also not be forgotten that many solvents are highly flammable and that fire is also a significant health hazard. The health effects of solvents are listed in Table 11.2.

Acute effects often involve the central nervous system, because of the rapid absorption of the solvent from the lungs and direct distribution to the brain. The immediate effects may result in mild impairment of judgment or drowsiness. In most situations these effects are not serious and will end quickly once exposure stops. In some circumstances a slight lapse of judgment could be disastrous. A person responding to a hazardous material spill or perhaps a fire must take appropriate precautions to limit exposure to any solvents that could impair judgment and thus increase risk of injury.

Chronic exposure to solvents can result in a range of organ system effects. Damage to the peripheral nervous system results in a tingling sensation and loss of feeling in the hands and feet, increased reaction time, and decreased coordination. Reproductive effects include decreased and damaged sperm causing a loss in fertility. Liver and kidney damage is possible from a range of solvents. Cancer is also caused by a number of different solvents, such as benzene and carbon tetrachloride.

There is no doubt that repeated exposure to high levels of solvent can result in permanent damage to the nervous system. These changes may result in impaired learning and memory, decreased attention span, and other psychological effects. There is also considerable data to indicate that chronic low-level exposure to solvents can result in a cluster of symptoms variously referred to as painter's syndrome, organic solvent syndrome, or chronic solvent encephalopathy. Painter's syndrome was first described in Scandinavia in the late 1970s and became a recognized occupational disease in these countries. The cluster of symptoms includes headache, fatigue, sleep disorders, personality changes, and emotional lability, progressing to impaired intellectual function and ultimately dementia. Early symptoms are often reversible if exposure is stopped.

The easy availability of solvents in commercial and household products combined with the rapid onset of nervous system effects encourages the use of solvents as an intoxicating drug. The recreational inhalation of solvents can produce euphoria, visual and auditory hallucinations, and sedation. As mentioned above, repeated exposure to high levels of solvents results in permanent brain damage. Beyond purposeful inhalation for the direct nervous system effects, there is accidental exposure. Children who accidentally drink furniture polish or other solvent-based household products are vulnerable to nervous system effects and possibly pneumonitis.

## 11.6 Reducing exposure

From a health perspective, there are few redeeming features of solvents except when used as anesthetics. Clearly the simple recommendation is to avoid exposure unless administered for some medical reason. In the workplace, appropriate ventilation and personal safety equipment should be in place at all times. There are numerous national and international regulations on solvent exposure in the workplace. Substitution of less-toxic solvents in processes and products can reduce the risk of injury.

## 11.7 Regulatory standards

In the workplace, standards and exposure recommendation are complex because they must address both level and duration of exposure. Below are some of the common terms used in establishing exposure recommendations.

- STEL – short-term exposure limits (15 minute exposure) – protect against acute effects – protect against loss of consciousness or loss of performance – need for short-term exposure in emergency situation
- TLV – threshold limit value
- TLV-C – threshold limit value-C (ceiling not to be exceeded)
- TWA – time-waited average (acceptable for 8 hour per day, 40 hour per week)

## 11.8 Recommendation and conclusions

Solvents are common around the home and workplace. As with most toxic substances, the best policy is to substitute less toxic products whenever possible, and reduce exposure via ventilation or protective equipment if substitutes are not available. Inhalation of solvents is particularly dangerous because of the rapid exchange in the lungs and quick access to the nervous system. Solvent inhalation produces predictable short-term effects but the long-term effects of repeated solvent exposure are not well characterized.

## 11.9 More information and references

### 11.9.1 Slide presentation

- A Small Dose of Solvents presentation material. Online. Available HTTP: <http://www.crcpress.com/e_products/> and follow the links to downloads and then the catalog number TF1691.
  Web site contains presentation material on the health effects of solvents.

### 11.9.2 European, Asian, and international agencies

■  United Nations Office for Drug Control and Crime Prevention (UN ODCCP). Online. Available HTTP: <http://www.undcp.org/odccp/index.html> (accessed: 9 April 2003).

### 11.9.3 North American agencies

■  US Department of Labor – Occupational Safety & Health Administration (OSHA). Online. Available HTTP: <http://www.osha.gov/SLTC/solvents/index.html> (accessed: 9 April 2003).
   This site has extensive information on solvents in the workplace.
■  US Agency for Toxic Substance Disease Registry (ATSDR). Online. Available HTTP: <http://www.atsdr.cdc.gov/toxfaq.html> (accessed: 9 April 2003).
   Site contains fact sheets and case studies on many common solvents.
■  US National Institute on Drug Abuse (NIDA). Online. Available HTTP: <http://www.nida.nih.gov/DrugPages/> (accessed: 9 April 2003).
   Site contains information on inhalants as drugs of abuse.
■  US Environmental Protection Agency (EPA) Integrated Solvent Substitution Data System. Online. Available HTTP: <http://es.epa.gov/issds/> (accessed: 9 April 2003).
   Site has comprehensive information on alternatives to solvents for products and processes.

### 11.9.4 Non-government organizations

■  The Wood Library–Museum of Anesthesiology. Online. Available HTTP: <http://www.asahq.org/wlm/homepage.html> (accessed: 9 April 2003).
   The objective of the Wood Library–Museum of Anesthesiology is to collect and preserve literature and equipment pertaining to anesthesiology and to make available to the anesthesiology community, others in the medical profession and the public the most comprehensive educational, scientific, and archival resources in anesthesiology
■  Anesthesia Nursing & Medicine. Online. Available HTTP: <http://www.anesthesia-nursing.com/> (accessed: 9 April 2003).
   Site has in-depth information on the history and current practice of anesthesia.

### 11.9.5 References

■  Charles Darwin (1993). The Autobiography of Charles Darwin 1809–1882, Nora Barlow (ed.), W. W. Norton & Company, New York, NY, 253 pp.
■  MMWR. (2001). n-Hexane-related peripheral neuropathy among automotive technicians – California, 1999–2000. Vol 50, No 45;1011, 11/16/2001. Online. Available HTTP: <http://www.cdc.gov/mmwr/PDF/wk/mm5045.pdf> (accessed: 9 April 2003).

# Chapter 12

# Radiation

## Contents

- Dossier – nonionizing radiation
- Dossier – ionizing radiation
- Case studies
- Introduction and history
- Biological and physical properties
- Health effects
- Reducing exposure
- Regulatory standards
- Recommendation and conclusions
- More information and references

### 12.1 Dossier – nonionizing radiation

**Use:** power transmission, communication, illumination, heating, cooking, vision, photosynthesis (sunlight), etc.

**Source:** Ultraviolet light, visible light, infrared radiation, microwaves, radio and TV, power transmission

**Recommended exposure:** different depending on source, i.e. sunlight can damage skin

**Absorption:** depends on source

**Sensitive individuals:** variable, i.e. fair-skinned children (sunburn)

Toxicity/symptoms: Depends on source. Solar radiation: sunburn, cataracts, cancer; microwave radiation: warming of skin or internal organs, controversy exists around exposure to low frequency energy such as AC power lines.
Regulatory facts: government regulates exposure
General facts: long history of use
Environmental: Our dependency on energy results in a range of consequences, for example drilling for oil and mining coal to run power plants to generate electricity, in turn mercury is released in the atmosphere from burning coal
Recommendations: depending on individual sensitivity; limit exposure to solar radiation (ultraviolet radiation); reduce energy consumption

## 12.2 Dossier – ionizing radiation

Use: nuclear power, medical X-rays, medical diagnostics, scientific research, cancer treatment, cathode ray tube displays
Source: radon, X-rays, radioactive materials produce alpha, beta, and gamma radiation, cosmic rays from the sun and space
Recommended daily intake: none (not essential)
Absorption: interaction with atoms of tissue
Sensitive individuals: children, developing organisms
Toxicity/symptoms: damages DNA leading to cancer
Regulatory facts: heavily regulated
General facts: long history of exposure to low levels
Environmental: many clean-up sites form radioactive waste
Recommendations: limit exposure

## 12.3 Case studies

### 12.3.1 Radium girls

"Not to worry," their bosses told them. "If you swallow any radium, it'll make your cheeks rosy."

The women at Radium Dial sometimes painted their teeth and faces and then turned off the lights for a laugh.

Martha Irvine, *Radium Girls*, Associated Press, Buffalo News, 1998.

Marie Curie discovered radium in her laboratory in Paris in 1898. The unique properties of this naturally occurring radioactive element suggested to many that it had therapeutic uses. In the early 1900s, radium therapy was accepted by the American Medical Association. Radium was thought to cure a range of illnesses including arthritis, stomach ailments, and cancer. Tonics of radium were available for oral consumption, to "bring the sun to your stomach", as well as by injection. In reality, the alpha particle emissions of radium caused rather than cured cancer.

This cancer-causing effect of radium was realized only after the tragic plight of young women working as radium dial painters came to the public's attention. The use of radium on watch dials began before the First World War and continued during the 1920s. The US Radium Corporation employed young women to paint radium on watch dials. The women used their lips to point the brushes. Each time they pointed their brushes, they ingested a small amount of radium. The radium moved to the bone where it continued to emit alpha radiation. The alpha radiation damaged the cells near the radium particle. As a result of their exposure to radium, many of these women developed painfully debilitating bone decay and died of cancer. The long half-life of radium combined with it being sequestered in the bone resulted in a lifetime of radiation exposure. During the 1920s, a group of these women sued the Radium Corporation. Many of them were victorious in court and received a small amount of money, becoming the first to receive compensation for occupational injury. It is estimated that 4000 people, mostly women, were occupationally exposed to radium as watch dial painters. This population formed the basis of several studies into the long-term effects of radiation. Their story was made into the movie *Radium City* (1987) and more recently a play. There is also an excellent book entitled *Radium Girls: Women and Industrial Health Reform, 1910–1935* by Claudia Clark.

### 12.3.2 Solar radiation – sunlight from warmth to sunburn

Sunlight is essential for life, but as with most things, too much can be harmful. The World Health Organization estimates that 2 to 3 million non-malignant skin cancers and over 130,000 malignant melanomas occur globally each year. Ultraviolet (UV) radiation is the primary cause of skin cancer as well as many more acute cases of sunburn. Thinning of the atmospheric ozone layer, which filters much of the UV radiation, has increased the harmful effects of elevated UV exposure. UV exposure can increase the incidence of cataracts of the eye, reduce the effectiveness of the immune system, and accelerate the effects of aging. Skin damage is also common, particularly for fair-skinned people exposed to too much UV radiation from the sun. Children need additional protection from the sun because their skin is more sensitive to the effects of UV radiation. Sunlight is necessary, however, because it stimulates the synthesis of vitamin D, which is important in the metabolism of calcium.

Solar radiation is part of the electromagnetic spectrum of radiation. The wavelength of visible light is 400–760 nanometers (nm), less than 400 nm is ultraviolet (UV) radiation and greater than 760 nm is infrared radiation, the heat of the sun. Our skin, the largest organ of the body, has naturally developed means to protect us from UV radiation. UV radiation stimulates the production of the melanin pigment, which absorbs UV radiation and protects the skin cells from damage. People with darker colored skin have ongoing production of melanin and are better protected from damage than people with less skin color. There is considerable genetic variation in the production of melanin. Sunburn occurs when UV radiation damages a cell and the body responds by increasing blood flow, resulting in a reddish and hot presentation. UV radiation damages cellular DNA. Although the cells have built-in repair mechanisms, repeated DNA damage can result in skin cancer.

Chemicals in sunscreens work much like melanin to absorb UV radiation. The most common is para-aminobenzoic acid or PABA, but there are others. Most glass, but not clear plastic, will block UV radiation. Relatively simple measures, such as hats and clothing, will greatly reduce exposure. About 90% of UV radiation is reflected by snow, making snow blindness a significant concern.

UV radiation illustrates the basic principles of toxicology in that individual sensitivity varies greatly, and it is best to limit your dose (exposure) to control your response. The challenge is to understand and manage the risk and benefits of our individual exposure and resulting acute and long-term effects.

## 12.4 Introduction and history

All life is dependent on small doses of electromagnetic radiation. Plants depend on small doses of radiation, living by converting this energy through photosynthesis to sustain them and in turn provide food for animals. We are surrounded by and depend on radiation-emitting devices, from the sun to our cell phones and radios, from medical X-rays to the electricity that powers our homes. There are many benefits from radiation-emitting devices, but we are still learning about some of the health effects. To explore the health effects of radiation exposure effectively, it is first necessary to examine the physics of radiation.

The electromagnetic spectrum is roughly divided into ionizing and nonionizing radiation (Figure 12.1). The distinction depends on the amount of energy carried by the radiation, which is directly related to the frequency of vibration of the electric and magnetic fields. When the frequency (and hence energy) is high enough, the radiation can separate electrons from atoms, ionizing the material it passes through. Nonionizing radiation includes ultraviolet, visible, infrared, microwaves, radio and TV, and power transmission. We depend on the sun's radiation for photosynthesis and heat. Ionizing radiation includes high-energy radiation such as cosmic rays,

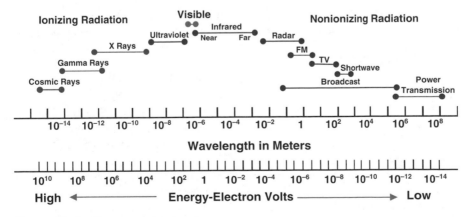

**Figure 12.1.** Electromagnetic spectrum.

X-rays, or gamma rays generated by nuclear decay. Ionizing radiation also includes several types of subatomic particles, such as beta radiation (high-energy electrons) and alpha radiation (helium ions) and others. Medical X-rays are an example of a common beneficial exposure to ionizing radiation. Nuclear radiation is used to generate electricity and cure disease, but is also an important element in military weapons. Uses of nuclear radiation pose serious issues of human exposure and environmental contamination.

The understanding and subsequent use of various forms of radiation provide a fascinating window into human civilization. The cave dwellers were probably the first to manage radiation when they learned to control and use fire. The control and use of electricity was another huge step forward. But the turn of the twentieth century really marked the beginning of rapid progress in the understanding and harnessing of the power of radiation. This period also ushered in a growing understanding of the potential adverse effects of radiation exposure. In 1903, Marie Curie and Pierre Curie, along with Henri Becquerel, were awarded the Nobel Prize in physics for their contributions to understanding radioactivity, including the properties of uranium. To this day, the "curie" and the "becquerel" are used as units of measure in radiation studies. In 1895, Wilhem Conrad Roentgen discovered X-rays, and in 1901 he was awarded the first Nobel Prize for physics. These discoveries led to significant advances in medicine. Work by Enrico Fermi and others led to the first sustained nuclear chain reaction in a laboratory beneath the University of Chicago football stadium on 2 December 1942. Subsequently, this knowledge was used to develop the atomic bombs that were dropped on Japan in an effort to end the Second World War. Much of our understanding of the effects of nuclear radiation exposure has come from the victims in Japan as well as the many workers in uranium mines.

## 12.5 Biological and physical properties

### 12.5.1 Nonionizing radiation

Nonionizing radiation has less energy and, in general, is less interactive with biological material than ionizing radiation. We are surrounded by energy from devices and products that emit nonionizing radiation. For example, radio and TV transmission surround us but do not significantly interact with our bodies. Light bulbs convert electrical energy into visible light and heat, all forms of nonionizing radiation.

On the other hand, a microwave oven is designed to interact with biological material to produce heat. The microwave energy readily passes through paper, glass, and plastic but is absorbed by water molecules in food, causing them to vibrate, which heats the material. The microwave oven generates enough energy to be potentially harmful if there was not appropriate shielding. Government regulations are in place to limit the amount of energy leakage from microwave ovens. Note that the interaction of microwaves with human tissue is not through ionization but rather heating.

Around our home we are exposed to a variety of different types of radiation. Home appliances such as hair dryers emit electromagnetic radiation. Our TVs and computer monitors expose us to additional electromagnetic radiation, as do our cell phones and radios (Table 12.1).

### Table 12.1 Products that depend on nonionizing radiation

Cellular phones
Cellular telephone base stations
Radio towers
Microwave towers
Lasers (including laser pointers)
Magnetic resonance imaging (MRI)
Radio transmissions (am or fm)
TV transmissions
Short-wave radio transmissions
Satellite transmissions
Electrical blankets
Appliances
Light bulbs
Computer and TV monitors
Microwave ovens
Power lines (both large and small)
Visible light
Ultraviolet radiation
Radar

## 12.5.2 Ionizing radiation

Ionizing radiation has sufficient energy to produce ion pairs as it passes through matter, that is, it frees electrons and leaves the rest of the atoms positively charged. In other words, there is enough energy to remove an electron from an atom. The energy released is enough to break bonds in DNA, which can lead to significant cellular damage and cancer. The health effects and dose–response relationship for radiation exposure are well established from human exposures to radiation and other research. The four main types of ionizing radiation are alpha particles, beta particles (electrons), gamma rays, and X-rays.

Alpha particles are heavy in weight and relatively low energy emissions from the nucleus of radioactive material. The transfer of energy occurs over a very short distance of about 10 cm in air. A piece of paper or layer of skin will stop an alpha particle. The primary hazard is from internal exposure to an alpha-emitting material. Cells close to the alpha particle-emitting material will be damaged. Typical sites of accumulation include bone, kidney, liver, lung, and spleen. Radium is an alpha particle emitter that when ingested accumulates in the bone, causing a bone sarcoma.

Airplane travel can increase our exposure to cosmic and solar radiation that is normally blocked by the atmosphere. Radiation intensity is greater across the poles and at higher altitudes, thus individual exposure varies depending on the route of travel. Storms on the sun can produce solar flares that can release larger amounts of radiation than normal. For the occasional traveler this radiation exposure is well below recommended limits established by regulatory authorities. However, frequent

### Table 12.2 Measures of radiation energy

| Item | Previous unit | SI unit | Ratios |
|------|---------------|---------|--------|
| Activity | curie (Ci) | bequerel (Bq) | $1\ Ci = 3.7 \times 10^{10}\ Bq$<br>$1\ mCi = 37\ MBq$<br>$1\ \mu Ci = 37\ KBq$ |
| Exposure | roentgen (R) | X (coul/kg) | $1\ R = 2.58 \times 10^{-4}\ coul/kg$ |
| Absorbed dose | rad | gray (Gy)<br>Gy = 1 J/kg | $1\ Gy = 100\ rad$<br>$1\ rad = 10\ mGy$ |
| Equivalent dose | rem | sievert (Sv) | $1\ Sv = 100\ rem$<br>$1\ rem = 10\ mSv$ |

m = milli = 1/1000.

fliers and airline workers can be exposed to levels of radiation that exceed established guidelines.

Sources of ionizing radiation or exposed populations:

- Medical X-ray devices (patients, medical workers)
- Radioactive material producing alpha, beta, and gamma radiation (laboratory workers, hospital workers, patients)
- Cosmic rays from the sun and space (airplane travelers)

### 12.5.3 Radiation units

The units used to describe exposure and dose of ionizing radiation to living material are confusing, at best. First, the units have changed to an international system, SI, which stands for Systeme Internationale. We will use the SI system, but Table 12.2 compares the SI system with the older system.

The fundamental descriptive unit of ionizing radiation is the amount of energy, expressed in coulombs per kilogram of air, and is the unit of exposure in air. The absorbed dose is the amount of energy absorbed by a specific material such as the human body and is described as the gray (Gy), previously the rad. The energy transfer of the different particles and gamma rays is different. A weighting fact is used to allow comparison between these different energy transfers. The unit for the equivalent dose is the sievert (Sv). A further refinement is possible that applies a weighting fact to each type of tissue. Recommended limits on radiation exposure are expressed in Sv.

### 12.6 Health effects

We are constantly exposed to ionizing and nonionizing radiation from naturally occurring sources as well as radiation generated and managed by our society. The challenge is to understand and manage the risk and benefits of our individual exposure.

### 12.6.1 Nonionizing radiation

We are surrounded by nonionizing radiation, the majority of which does us no harm. The visible light from the sun, the light bulbs in our homes, radio and TV transmissions, and electric appliances all contribute to our background exposure to nonionizing radiation. Most evidence indicates that this radiation is harmless, although some studies have found possible effects. However, at higher levels and longer durations of exposure, nonionizing radiation can be harmful.

The classic example is sunlight or solar radiation. Ultraviolet radiation from the sun, the part of the electromagnetic spectrum with a wavelength less than 400 nm, can damage the skin. Sunburn (erythema) is the result of excessive exposure of our skin to UV radiation when we lack the protection of UV-absorbing melanin (see case study above). Acute cellular damage causes an inflammatory-type response and increased vascular circulation (vasodilation) close to the skin. The increased circulation causes the redness and hot feeling to the skin. Lightly pressing on the skin pushes the blood away and the spot appears white. Darker skinned people have an ongoing production of melanin, which protects them to some extent from UV radiation. In lighter skinned people, UV radiation stimulates the production of melanin, producing a tan and protection against UV radiation. Extreme exposure can result in blistering and severe skin damage. UV radiation can also damage cellular DNA. Repeated damage can overwhelm the DNA repair mechanism, resulting in skin cancer. Skin cancer accounts for approximately one-third of all cancers diagnosed each year. Thinning of the atmospheric ozone layer, which filters UV radiation, is suspected as being one cause of the increased incidence of skin cancer. Wearing protective clothing can reduce UV radiation exposure. Sunscreen lotions contain a chemical that absorbs the UV radiation in a similar manner to melanin. Solar radiation is a classic example of the principles of toxicology: beware of individual sensitivity and dose yourself in a way that limits any adverse response.

The use of microwave and radiofrequency (MW/RF) devices has grown dramatically in the past 20 years. The most popular consumer products are microwave ovens and cell or mobile phones. MW/RF radiation is also used in a wide range of commercial applications such as radar, solder machines, welders, heat sealers, drying equipment, glue curing, and others. In biological tissues, microwave radiation produces heat. A warming sensation can be felt on the skin or even internal organs and body temperature can be raised. Microwave ovens must comply with government standards to minimize exposure. Cell phones use low-level radiofrequency energy that is well below a level that would warm tissue, but there is ongoing research in effects related to chronic exposure. In the United States, the Food and Drug Administration is responsible for protecting the public from radiation from microwave ovens, television sets, computer monitors, and cell phones.

### 12.6.2 Ionizing radiation

Ionizing radiation is more harmful that nonionizing radiation, because it has enough energy to remove an electron from an atom and thus directly damage biological material. The energy is enough to damage DNA, which can result in cell death or cancer. The study of ionizing radiation is a large area of classical toxicology, which has produced a tremendous understanding of the dose–response relationship of exposure. The primary effect of ionizing radiation is cancer. It can also affect the developing fetus of mothers exposed during pregnancy. Radiation exposure has a direct dose–response relationship: the more radiation you receive, the greater your chance of developing cancer.

Our knowledge of the effects of radiation developed gradually from tragic experience over the last century. Early in the century, researchers such as Marie Curie died of cancer, presumably related to her radiation exposure. At the time some writers even extolled the virtues of people dying to advance the cause of science. Occupational exposure was another tragic learning environment. Young women employed to paint radium on watch dials died from bone cancer in the 1920s and 1930s (see above case study). During this time radium was promoted as a cure for many maladies and even recognized by the American Medical Association. We had a lot to learn.

From uranium mineworkers we learned of the hazards of radon exposure. Radon is a radioactive gas that is present in the uranium mines, as well as in high concentration in the soil in some places. Radon exposure results in lung and esophageal cancer. The actual carcinogens are daughter products of radon that adhere to the internal tissue and emit alpha particles. While excess cancer in mineworkers is well established, there is considerable concern about the effects of lower level chronic exposure that might be found in the home, particularly in the basement (see chapter on cancer and genetic toxicology).

A great deal was learned from the atomic bomb survivors. The US military dropped the first atomic bomb on Hiroshima, Japan on 6 August 1945 and a second on Nagasaki, Japan, three days later. The bombs used two different types of radioactive material, $^{235}U$ in the first bomb and $^{239}Pu$ in the second. It is estimated that 64,000 people died from the initial blast and radiation exposure. Approximately 100,000 survivors were enrolled in follow-up studies, which confirmed an increased incidence of cancer.

X-rays were also used to treat disease. From 1905 to 1960, X-rays were used to treat ringworm in children. Well into the 1950s, X-rays were used to treat a degenerative bone disease called ankylosing spondylitis.

The primary lesson learned in all these examples is that the greater the dose, the greater the likelihood of developing cancer. The second lesson was that there could be a very long delay in the onset of the cancer, from 10 to 40 years. It should be remembered that we evolved with a background exposure to naturally occurring ionizing radiation, and we continue to be exposed to low levels of natural background radiation. Some have estimated that 1 in 100 cancers are the result of this background exposure

## 12.7 Reducing exposure

Three ways to reduce exposure to radiation are:

- Time – Limit the amount of time you spend near the source of radiation. One of the easiest examples is that you avoid getting sunburned by limiting the amount of time in bright sunlight. This same principle applies to ionizing radiation such as a radioactive material.

- Distance – Increase your distance from the source of radiation. Emissions from the source of radiation decrease in intensity rapidly.
- Shielding – The effectiveness of shielding depends on the type of radiation, but in general placing absorbent shielding material between you and the radiation source reduces exposure. This can be as simple as wearing a hat to protect your face from the sun or using a lead apron in the dentist's chair to shield other parts of your body from the dental X-rays.

## 12.8 Regulatory standards

The first organized effort to protect people from radiation exposure began in 1915 when the British Roentgen Society adopted a resolution to protect people from X-rays.

In 1922 the United States adopted the British protection rules and various government and nongovernmental groups were formed to protect people from radiation. In 1959, the Federal Radiation Council was formed to advise the president and recommend standards. In 1970, the US Environmental Protection Agency was formed and took over these responsibilities. Now several government agencies are responsible for protecting people from radiation-emitting devices.

### 12.8.1 Standards for radiation exposure

Recommended exposure limits are set by the US National Council on Radiation Protection (NCRP) and worldwide by the International Council on Radiation Protection (ICRP). The occupational exposure guidelines are 100 mSv in 5 years (average, 20 mSv per year) with a limit of 50 mSv in any single year. For the general public, the standard is 1 mSv per year. This must be put in the context of natural background radiation, which is approximately 3 mSv/year depending upon location (such as elevation) as well as other variables.

## 12.9 Recommendation and conclusions

We evolved in an environment of natural radiation from the solar energy of the sun to radioactive elements. Radiation is described by the electromagnetic spectrum in terms of wavelength and frequency. A further division is made between ionizing and nonionizing radiation. Ionizing radiation has sufficient energy to remove electrons, thus the ability to damage biological tissue directly. During the past century we have learned how to exploit the electromagnetic spectrum for many useful purposes (and some not so useful) and along the way learned about some of the hazards of radiation exposure.

Some radiation is helpful and necessary, as in the case of sunlight, which allows us to see the world. The nonionizing radiation of the sun warms us, but too much ultraviolet radiation can cause sunburn or cancer depending on our individual sensitivity. There is clearly a dose – response relationship between exposure and effect, with individual sensitivity playing an important role. Microwave and radiofrequency radiation are incredibly useful in heating and transmitting information.

Ionizing radiation is far more dangerous than nonionizing radiation because it can directly damage cellular DNA and proteins, causing cell death or possibly cancer.

Ionizing radiation is divided into alpha and beta particles and gamma rays. Each has its unique characteristics, which require different safety approaches. In general, the more radiation exposure a person receives, the greater the likelihood of cancer.

## 12.10 More information and references

### 12.10.1 Slide presentation

■ A Small Dose of Radiation presentation material. Online. Available HTTP: <http://www.crcpress.com/e_products/> and follow the links to downloads and then the catalog number TF1691.
Web site contains presentation material on the health effects of radiation.

### 12.10.2 European, Asian, and international agencies

■ Australian Radiation Protection and Nuclear Safety Agency (ARPANSA). Online. Available HTTP: <http://www.arpansa.gov.au/> (accessed: 9 April 2003). (ARPANSA) is "charged with responsibility for protecting the health and safety of people, and the environment, from the harmful effects of ionizing and non-ionizing radiation".
■ England – Department of Health – Committee on Medical Aspects of Radiation in the Environment (COMPARE). Online. Available HTTP: <http://www.doh.gov.uk/comare/comare.htm> (accessed: 9 April 2003). COMPARE is "responsible for assessing and advising agencies on the health effects of natural and man-made radiation in the environment".
■ World Health Organization (WHO). Online. Available HTTP: <http://www.who.int/health_topics/ultraviolet_rays/en/> (accessed: 9 April 2003). Site contains information on the global efforts to reduce UV radiation exposure.

### 12.10.3 North American agencies

■ Health Canada – Radiation Protection. Online. Available HTTP: <http://www.hc-sc.gc.ca/hecs-sesc/ccrpb/index.htm> (accessed: 9 April 2003). Health Canada provides information on the health effects of radiation for consumer and clinical radiation protection.
■ US Centers for Disease Control and Prevention (CDC) National Center for Environmental Health. Online. Available HTTP: <http://www.cdc.gov/nceh/> (accessed: 9 April 2003). This site contains information on health effects and emergency response to radiation exposure.
■ US Environmental Protection Agency (EPA). Online. Available HTTP: <http://www.epa.gov/radiation/> (accessed: 9 April 2003). This site has a tremendous amount of information on ionizing and nonionizing radiation and environmental contamination.
■ US Environmental Protection Agency (EPA) What Is Your Annual Radiation Dose? Online. Available HTTP: <http://www.epa.gov/radiation/students/calculate.html> (accessed: 9 April 2003).

This site shows you how to examine your current exposure to radiation.

- US Food and Drug Administration – Center for Devices and Radiological Health. Online. Available HTTP: <http://www.fda.gov/cdrh/comp/eprc.html> (accessed: 9 April 2003).
  This site contains information on the health effects and regulation of radiation-emitting devices and products. "Protecting the public health by providing reasonable assurance of the safety and effectiveness of medical devices and by eliminating unnecessary human exposure to radiation emitted from electronic products."

- US Food and Drug Administration – Cell Phone Facts. Online. Available HTTP: <http://www.fda.gov/cellphones/qa.html#22> (accessed: 9 April 2003).
  Site contains general and regulatory information on cell phones and related technology.

- US Federal Communications Commission – Office of Engineering and Technology – Radio Frequency Safety. Online. Available HTTP: <http://www.fcc.gov/oet/rfsafety/> (accessed: 9 April 2003).

- US Department of Labor, Occupational Safety & Health Administration (OSHA), Radiofrequency/Microwave Radiation. Online. Available HTTP: <http://www.osha-slc.gov/SLTC/radiofrequencyradiation/index.html> (accessed: 9 April 2003).
  The OSHA site contains information on microwave and radiofrequency devices.

- US New Jersey – Nonionizing Radiation Section. Online. Available HTTP: <http://www.state.nj.us/dep/rpp> (accessed: 9 April 2003).
  New Jersey has a wide range of information on radiation.

- US Agency for Toxic Substance Disease Registry (ATSDR). Online. Available HTTP: <http://www.atsdr.cdc.gov/> (accessed: 9 April 2003).
  See toxicology fact sheets Tox FAQs™ and case studies in environmental health.

- US Department of Commerce, National Oceanic and Atmospheric Administration (NOAA), Air Resources Laboratory. Online. Available HTTP: <http://www.arl.noaa.gov/> (accessed: 9 April 2003).
  Site contains UV radiation monitoring information for the US.

- US Nuclear Regulatory Commission (NRC). Online. Available HTTP: <http://www.nrc.gov/> (accessed: 9 April 2003).
  "The NRC regulates US commercial nuclear power plants and the civilian use of nuclear materials."

### 12.10.4 Non-government organizations

- National Council on Radiation Protection and Measurements (NCRP). Online. Available HTTP: <http://www.ncrp.com/> (accessed: 9 April 2003). "The NCRP seeks to formulate and widely disseminate information, guidance and recommendations on radiation protection and measurements which represent the consensus of leading scientific thinking."
- Health Physics Society. Online. Available HTTP: <http://www.hps.org/> (accessed: 9 April 2003).
  Site has extensive information about health physics and radiation protection.

- University of Michigan – Radiation & Health Physics. Online. Available HTTP: <http://www.umich.edu/~radinfo/> (accessed: 9 April 2003).
  Site contains information "written for three distinct groups: the General Public, Students and the Health Physics community at large".

### 12.10.5 References

- *Radium Girls: Women and Industrial Health Reform, 1910–1935* by Claudia Clark, Publisher: University of North Carolina Pr; ISBN: 0807823317; (June 1997), 384 pp.

# Chapter 13

## Animal and plant toxins

## Contents

### 13.1 Dossier – animal toxins

**Name:** animal venoms and poisons
**Use:** medicinal uses
**Source:** spiders, insects, snakes, lizards, fish, and frogs
**Recommended daily intake:** none (not essential)
**Absorption:** varies but can be very fast, e.g. bites
**Sensitive individuals:** children (small size), previously sensitized
**Toxicity/symptoms:** varies
**Regulatory facts:** none
**General facts:** long history of use and desire to avoid
**Environmental:** global distribution, concern about expanding distribution to new areas
**Recommendations:** avoid

### 13.2 Dossier – plant toxins

**Name:** plants
**Use:** medicinal uses
**Source:** wide variety of plants
**Recommended daily intake:** none (not essential)
**Absorption:** intestine, skin
**Sensitive individuals:** children (small size), previously sensitized
**Toxicity/symptoms:** varies
**Regulatory facts:** none
**General facts:** long history of use and desire to avoid
**Environmental:** global distribution, concern about expanding distribution to new areas
**Recommendations:** generally avoid

## 13.3 Case studies

### 13.3.1 Puffer fish

About 100 species of puffer fish use the powerful tetrodotoxin to discourage consumption by predators. Tetrodotoxin is found in all organs of the fish but is highest in liver, skin, and intestine. The origins of the toxin are not clear, but one possibility is that the fish come in contact with bacteria that produce tetrodotoxin. Puffer fish may also have elevated levels of saxitoxin, a neurotoxin responsible for paralysis in shellfish poisoning. Saxitoxin is produced by dinoflagellates (algae) and most often contaminates mussels, clams, and scallops. Both saxitoxin and tetrodotoxin are heat stable so cooking does not reduce toxicity. Tetrodotoxin causes paralysis by affecting sodium ion transport in both the central and peripheral nervous system. A low dose of tetrodotoxin produces tingling sensations and numbness around the mouth, fingers, and toes. Higher doses produce nausea, vomiting, respiratory failure, difficulty walking, extensive paralysis, and death. As little as 1 to 4 mg of the toxin can kill an adult. Saxitoxin has a very different chemical structure to tetrodotoxin, but similar effects on transport of cellular sodium; it produces similar neurological effects, but is less toxic that tetrodotoxin. Some people, particularly in Asia, consider the puffer fish a fine delicacy providing it is carefully prepared by experienced chiefs. The trick is to get just a small dose to feel mild tingling effects but not the more serious effects of the tetrodotoxin. In the United States tetrodotoxin poisoning is rare, but a recent report by the US CDC described several case studies of people catching and consuming puffer fish containing elevated levels of these toxins and suffering the ill effects (MMWR, 2002).

### 13.3.2 Jimson weed (thorn apple)

Jimson weed is the common name of one plant in a family of plants recognized since ancient times for their interesting effects on the nervous system. The deadly nightshade plant (*Atropa belladonna*) was used in the Roman Empire and during the Middle Ages both as a cure and a poison. Women used preparations from this plant to dilate their pupils as a sign of allure and beauty. Some say the name belladonna refers to beautiful Italian women with dilated pupils. The drug responsible for these effects is called atropine, from the other part of the scientific name for deadly nightshade. We are commonly given a form of atropine (homatropine) to dilate our pupils during eye examination. This is a short-acting form of atropine that keeps eyes dilated for a few hours rather than the seven or more days that results from atropine. Atropine is also the drug used to counteract the effects of pesticides and chemical warfare agents that act by inhibiting acetylcholinesterase. In addition to atropine, this family of plants contains scopolamine and other belladonna alkaloids. They act by inhibiting the actions of acetylcholine in the central and peripheral nervous systems. Besides dilation of the pupils, exposure to the belladonna alkaloids stops salivation, causing a dry mouth and difficulty swallowing, and produces an irregular heart rate. A larger dose causes central nervous system effects such as hallucinations, loss of memory, and confusion. Jimson weed, part of the belladonna family of plants, is a common weed in North America. The easy availability of jimson weed combined with its ability to alter the nervous system leads to youth experimentation with the plant. Unfortunately, the consequences, especially when combined with other drugs, can be very serious and even lead to death (MMWR, 1995).

### 13.3.3 Mushroom poisoning

Worldwide, the most dangerous mushrooms are the "death cap" mushroom (*Amanita phalloides*) and the "death angel" (*Amanita ocreata*). The greatest number of deaths occurs in children less than 10 years of age, but adults are also susceptible. Often it is difficult to associate symptoms with eating the mushrooms because there is a 10–12 hour delay before symptoms become apparent. The initial symptoms are nausea, vomiting, diarrhea, and irregular heart rate. Ultimately the toxin, amatoxin, damages the liver cells resulting in liver and kidney failure and possibly death. The amatoxin binds to RNA and inhibits protein synthesis. Amatoxin is very potent: ingestion of only 0.1 to 0.3 mg/kg of body weight results in death. For a child weighing 10 kg (or about 22 lbs) only 1 mg of amatoxin could result in a fatal poisoning. In 1997, the US CDC reported that 2 out of 4 people who picked and consumed the death angel mushroom died of liver failure. This report clearly demonstrates that care is necessary in consuming wild mushrooms (MMWR, 1997).

### 13.4 Introduction and history

The creatures of the world, both animals and plants, produce a wide range of biologically active substances. Biologically active substances produced by animals or plants that cause an adverse effect are called toxins. Toxins refers only to toxic agents produced by animals and plants, not toxic substances such a lead or pesticides. The classification of a substance as a toxin tends to be in the eye of the beholder. Is caffeine, a naturally occurring agent in many plants, a toxin or just a pharmacologically active compound or both?

The study of plant and animal toxins is truly fascinating. Toxins offer many lessons in dose–response as well as a window into the struggle for growth and survival in hostile environments. They are used offensively to aid in gathering food or defensively to ward off predictors. To accomplish these tasks, toxins must interact with biological tissue. The study of their biological activity has provided us with important drugs and greatly improved our understanding of the mechanisms of biology. Much of this work has only advanced since the 1970s, when the sensitive instrumentation necessary to separate these venomous mixtures became available. The toxins of the world are really the medicine chest of nature. Pharmaceutical companies explore the world looking for new plants or animals that might be producing a new drug naturally. We have come to depend upon many of the substances produced by animals and plants. On the other hand, we all learn to avoid the sting of bees, and we know that even some of our houseplants are toxic. Mushrooms are a classic example of species that can be good to eat, deadly poisons, or, when used judiciously, produce hallucinations that some find desirable. Foxglove and lily-of-the-valley contain a compound called digitalis that lowers blood pressure and prevents heart attacks. On the other hand, digitalis is quite toxic and the plants themselves are considered poisonous.

In the following sections we can only take a brief look at this fascinating subject.

## 13.5 Animal toxins

Animal toxins are roughly divided into venoms and poisons. Venoms are offensive, used in the quest for food. Snakes produce toxins that can immobilize or kill prey for food. The venom of spiders paralyzes insects to allow the spider to feed on the victim's body fluids. While the venoms may also be used defensively, their primary purpose is in the quest for food. Most venom is delivered from the mouth, as in snakes and spiders, but there are exceptions like the scorpion that uses its tail.

Poisons are primarily defensive, designed as protection against predators. Poisons are often sprayed or delivered with a stinger to penetrate the skin. Some fishes, for example, have poisonous spines. Toxins can also be on the skin or be part of the meat of the animal, thus making them poisonous to touch or eat. Some poisonous animals develop very colorful markings to advertise their undesirable qualities.

The purpose of the venom is offensive while that of a poison is defensive, which in turn influences the characteristics of the toxin. Venoms, either large or small molecules, are usually variants of essential biological molecules such as lipids, steroids, histamines or other proteins. They are often mixtures with a specific mechanism of action such as paralyzing the nervous system. Poisons are designed to teach a predator that this is not a good meal. They usually cause more localized pain to discourage a predator, but depending on the dose and sensitivity of the individual, the poison can be deadly.

There are some unique challenges for animals that produce toxin, particularly venoms. The toxin must be concentrated and stored in large enough dose to be effective but without being toxic to the animal that produces it. After a quick delivery, the toxin must be rapidly absorbed and act quickly to defeat that prey's response. Many toxins are the envy of the drug developers.

### 13.5.1 Arthropods

Insects, spiders, scorpions, crabs, centipedes, millipedes, and even some plankton are arthropods, the largest and most diverse animal phylum. Some are capable of producing very powerful toxins as an aid in the quest for food. Humans come in contact with these toxins, usually by accident or as a result of the animal defending itself. Some insects, mosquitoes and ticks for example, are capable of transmitting other organisms to humans that cause disease. While these organisms may be toxic to humans, they are not toxins and will not be discussed in this chapter.

#### 13.5.1.1 Arachnids (scorpions, spiders, ticks)

*Scorpions*

There are approximately 1000 species of scorpions but only around 75 are clinically important. In some parts of the world, scorpion stings are common and for the most part treated like bee or wasp stings, producing no long-lasting effects. There are a few scorpions with venom potent enough to harm humans, particularly children. The most potent venoms are low molecular weight proteins that affect the nervous system. There is usually immediate pain at the site of the sting, with elevated or irregular heart rate one of the first clinical signs. Most adults recover within 12 hours, but, because of their low weight, children are vulnerable to more serious and long-lasting clinical effects.

*Spiders*

Spiders use their venom to paralyze prey while they feast on the victim's body fluids. They primarily feed on insects and other spiders. The venom of about 200 out of the 30,000 species of spiders represents a risk to humans. The venom of spiders is a complex mixture of neuroactive proteins and other chemicals. Researchers have studied venoms both to understand the mechanism of their effects and in search of new drugs. If spiders were bigger they would be truly dangerous. Fortunately they are small, with only a very small amount of venom. Because of our much larger size we receive only a small dose, but when a spider bites another insect it delivers a very large dose indeed.

In the United States one of the infamous venomous spiders is the black widow spider, but there are many similar species found around the world in temperate and tropical climates. It has a number of common names depending on the region of the world and ranges in color from brown to gray to black. The black widow species is shiny black and on the belly of the females is a red hourglass. Both the male and female are venomous, but only the female has fangs large enough to penetrate human skin. The venom of this species is made up of large proteins thought to affect the transmission of calcium ions of nervous system cells. The initial sting of the bite is followed by muscle cramps, sweating, and possibly decreased blood pressure. There is no adequate treatment but the bite is seldom fatal.

Another globally distributed venomous spider is the brown or violin spider. It too comes in numerous varieties depending upon the region of the world. The spider has a range of colors but most unique are its six eyes. The venom of the brown recluse contains a range of proteins designed to dissolve the victim's cellular proteins, but the most active agent affects the red blood cells. The effects of the venom vary, but in the worst case there is serious necrosis of tissue at the center of the bite, with a surrounding area becoming red and swollen. The venom literally dissolves the cells of the skin and surrounding tissue, which of course triggers the body's own defensive reactions. Significant tissue damage can occur, particularly if the bite is on the face, but the bites are almost never fatal. There is no effective treatment for the venom other than supportive care.

The best protection is to avoid spider bites, especially those of dangerous spiders. It is important to recognize which kinds of spiders are potentially dangerous, since most are harmless and shouldn't be killed needlessly.

## Ticks

Ticks have a bad reputation for good reasons. Not only are they carriers of a number of diseases, the saliva of some can cause paralysis. North American natives were aware of tick paralysis, but the condition was officially noted as a disease of both animals and humans in 1912. The bites of at least 60 species of ticks can cause paralysis, which often does not appear until several days after the bite. The first indication is redness and swelling around the site of the bite. This is followed by neuromuscular weakness and difficulty in walking. If the tick is not removed, speech and breathing are affected, with eventual respiratory paralysis and death. Fortunately, removal of the tick results in a quick recovery of function. The exact mechanism of paralysis is not known but it appears to come from a substance that affects the neuromuscular junction. While not related to the venom of the tick saliva, the tick can also transmit diseases such as Lyme disease, Rocky Mountain spotted fever, Q fever, typhus, and others. Table 13.1 lists some venomous arachnids.

### Table 13.1 Venomous arachnids (scorpions, spiders, ticks)

| Class | Examples | Venom and delivery | Comments |
| --- | --- | --- | --- |
| Arachnids (scorpions, spiders, and ticks) | Scorpions | Stinger – neurotoxin, no enzymes | Localized pain, mostly dangerous to children |
| | Latrodectus – widow spiders (back, brown red-legged spider) | Bite – neurotoxin – large molecular proteins | Localized pain, sweating, muscle cramps, decreased blood pressure |
| | Loxosceles – brown or violin spiders | Bite – complex mixture of enzymes | Serious tissue damage and attacks blood cells |
| | Ticks | Bite – saliva neurotoxin – transmit other diseases | Tick paralysis – weakness and difficulty walking – remove tick |

## 13.5.1.2 Insects

Some moths and caterpillars produce irritating substances or fend off predators with substances that do not taste good and are thus avoided.

A much more aggressive group of insects, with great power for their size, that almost all of us have come in contact with are ants. Ants produce poisonous or irritating substances as a means of defense. Most ants have a stinger, and some can spray substances onto skin or the wound created by their powerful jaws. There are thousands of species of ants, and the poisonous substances they produce vary enormously. Some ants create substances with large amounts of protein that can cause an allergic response. Others ants produce formic acid which is very irritating to the skin. Fire ants, common in the United States, produce a substance rich in alkaloids, which can cause localized tissue destruction and necrosis. Multiple bites can be dangerous and even life threatening for both humans and animals. Multiple stings can cause nausea, vomiting, difficulty breathing, coma, and death.

---

**Bee stings**

A honey bee has about 150 μg of poison, but only a small fraction is typically injected. The faster the stinger is removed, the less the response.

---

The stings from bees, wasps, hornets, and related insects are well known to many people. Humans have collected honey for at least 6000 years. Honeybees sting when threatened and to protect their hive and honey from both humans and other predators, including wasps. Wasps are attracted to the smell of a hive's honey and will attempt to steal the honey. Watching the honeybees defend their hive from wasps illustrates their need for a stinger. The stinger of a honeybee is barbed and usually left behind in the skin, literally ripped out of a bee that will soon die. Left behind also is a complex substance of many different proteins including histamine, dopamine, and a substance that breaks down tissue. When stung, it is advisable to remove the stinger as soon as possible to reduce exposure. Some people advise putting a meat tenderizer on the site of the sting. This may help because a meat tenderizer is designed to digest protein and soften meat. In the event of a bee sting, the tenderizer is used to digest the bee protein. Response to bee stings varies enormously from almost nothing to life threatening. Usually there is localized swelling as the body rushes to wipe out the foreign protein that has invaded the body. Some people are highly allergic to bee stings (about 1 or 2 per 1000 people), and for them the response is not localized and results in a massive response that can lead to death. Even for those not allergic, multiple stings can cause breathing problems, decreased blood pressure, shock, and death.

Wasp stings tend to contain less protein and a more formic acid-type substance that produces an intense burning. Table 13.2 lists some poisonous and venomous insects.

**Table 13.2 Insects**

| Examples | Poison or venom | Comments |
| --- | --- | --- |
| Moths and caterpillars | Irritating substance | Designed so they do not taste good |
| Ants | Variable – proteins, formic acid and other | Variable response – irritation, allergic response, tissue damage |
| Honey bees | Complex proteins | Swelling, allergic reaction |
| Wasps | Formic acid | Irritating |

### 13.5.2 Reptiles

#### 13.5.2.1 Lizards

Humans are a far bigger threat to lizards than they are to us. Lizards are generally slow moving and nocturnal, with few enemies other than humans. The venom is a complex mixture that contains serotonin, a neurotransmitter, but lacks many of the other protein-degrading enzymes. Clinical effects are minor unless you are small and receive a large dose.

#### 13.5.2.2 Snakes

Snakes occupy a unique place in our collective imagination. The primary function of snake venom is to immobilize or kill prey for food. A secondary function of the venom is defensive or protective, but clearly snakes are not capable of eating large animals, such as humans. Often venomous snakes will strike but not release venom, which conserves a valuable resource. Approximately 400 of the more than 3500 species of snake are sufficiently venomous to be a threat to humans and other large animals.

Worldwide, there are an estimated 300,000 to 400,000 venomous snakebites per year with about 10% (or 30 000) resulting in death. In the United States, there are approximately 7000 venomous bites per year but only 1 in 500 deaths, testifying to the value of prompt medical treatment.

The most common venomous snakebites in North America are from vipers. This class of snakes has the most advanced venom delivery system. The venom is delivered through hinged tubular fangs that can be folded into the snake's mouth. The venom is quickly injected into the victim. The pit vipers, such as rattlesnakes, have a head sensor located between their nostril and eyes that is thought to guide the strike, even in the dark. The venom from vipers is a very complex enzymatic-based substance, which quickly causes localized swelling and tissue destruction (necrosis). The protein-based venom causes an allergic-type reaction leading to hemorrhage of body fluids, decreased blood pressure, shock, fluid in the lungs, and death.

The second most common venomous snakes are the Elapidae, of which cobras and coral snakes are well known. These snakes deliver their venom from fixed fangs and must hold onto the victim while the venom is released. These snakes tend to

### Table 13.3 Reptiles

| Class | Examples | Venom and delivery | Symptoms |
|---|---|---|---|
| Vipers (Viperidae) | Rattlesnakes Water moccasins Copperheads Bushmasters | Very complex enzymatic-based Advanced delivery – hinged tubular fangs | Swelling and necrosis at site, affects blood cells, hemorrhage, decreased blood pressure, shock |
| Elapidae | Cobras Kraits Coral snakes | Neurotoxin (some very potent) Fixed fangs, usually low dose | Nervous system effects, paralysis, numbness, respiratory failure |

be smaller than vipers and deliver a smaller dose of poison. But what they lack in size they make up for in potency. The venom of these snakes predominately affects the nervous system, causing paralysis and numbness. Death is usually the result of respiratory failure from nervous system effects. Table 13.3 lists some venomous snakes.

## 13.5.3 Marine animals

### 13.5.3.1 Shellfish

Shellfish such as mussels, clams, oysters, and scallops are not naturally toxic but can become so after feeding on plankton contaminated with a toxin. When visible, the blooming of the plankton (dinoflagellate) is called the red tide and can cause significant death among marine animals. There are several types of toxins, mostly affecting the nervous system. The newest, domoic acid, first appeared in 1987 off Prince Edward Island in Canada. This neurotoxin caused confusion and memory loss, particularly in the elderly. Several elderly people died following seizures and coma. Domoic acid is heat stable, so cooking does not affect the toxin. Government agencies now monitor for contaminants of shellfish and move quickly to restrict harvesting. The domoic acid incident clearly indicates the importance of ongoing monitoring of the food supply.

The puffer fish is probably the best known neurotoxic fish. Several related species of fish, as well as other marine life, such as some frogs, starfish, octopus, and others, contain tetrodotoxin. Many people consider this fish a delicacy despite the occasional death from poor preparation. Tetrodotoxin is heat stable but water soluble, so careful preparation is necessary to limit neurological effects. Symptoms of poisoning include a rapid onset of numbness in the lips and mouth, which then extends to the fingers and toes, followed by general weakness, dizziness, and respiratory failure, leading to death. The mechanism of action is similar to that of saxitoxin and affects sodium channel permeability.

It should also be remembered that fish high in the food chain, such as tuna, swordfish, and shark accumulate toxic substances like mercury or PCBs. Mercury affects the nervous system and is a proven reproductive hazard. Table 13.4 lists examples of marine animals that may be toxic.

### Table 13.4 Marine animals

| Animal class | Examples | Toxin | Symptoms | Comment |
|---|---|---|---|---|
| Shellfish (filter-feeding mollusks) | Mussels, clams, oysters, scallops | Several kinds of toxin taken up from plankton (dinoflagellate) | See below | |
| | Paralytic shellfish poisoning | Saxitoxin in their muscles | Numbness, respiratory paralysis | Sodium channel permeability |
| | Diarrheic shellfish poisoning | High molecular weight polyethers | Nausea, vomiting, diarrhea | Usually mild but annoying |
| | Neurotoxic shellfish poisoning | Brevetoxins | Numbness of mouth, muscular aches, dizziness | |
| | Amnesic shellfish poisoning | Domoic acid | Confusion, memory loss, seizure, coma | Affects elderly |
| Coelenterates | Jelly fish, anemona, coral | Nematocyst | Sting, muscle cramps | |
| Fish | Sea snail (cigua) and some fish, oysters and clams | Ciguatera, scaritoxin and maitotoxin | Numbness, salivation, cardiovascular effects, respiratory paralysis | Inhibits acetyl cholinesterase |
| Fish | Puffer fish (fugu) blowfish, toadfish . . . some frogs, starfish, ocopus | Tetrodotoxin | Nervous system numbness, paralysis, respiratory failure, death | Decreased sodium channel permeability |
| Fish | Tuna, shark, sword fish | Mercury | Neurotoxic, reproductive effects | |

## 13.6 Plant toxins

In the battle to survive, plants have developed a wide array of defensive measures. Plants produce a range of chemicals designed to fend off predators or discourage consumption by insects or animals. We will look at the chemicals that plants produce from a human prospective, that is, how they affect us when we eat or come in contact with the plant. For thousands of years humans have experimented with plants in a search for food, as treatment for illness, and even to alter one's perception of the world. Wide ranges of drugs are derived from plants, and the search continues by the world's leading pharmaceutical companies. Others promote the use of plants as herbal or natural medicine. This section will focus only on the toxicity of some of the better-known plants, organized by organ system affected.

Tables 13.5 to 13.10 below summarize the most important facts. The text provides additional information only if necessary to clarify a particular point. We can only scratch the surface of this fascinating area of biology.

**Table 13.5 Effects on skin**

| Organ system | Symptoms | Plant examples | Toxin/comment |
|---|---|---|---|
| Skin | Allergic dermatitis – plant<br>Rashes, itchy skin | Philodendron, poison ivy, cashew, bulbs of daffodils, hyacinths, tulips | Antibody mediated after initial sensitization, very variable response. Allergens located on outer cells of plant |
| | Allergic dermatitis – pollen<br>Sniffing and sneezing, runny eyes | Ragweed (North America), mugwort (Europe), grasses | Antibody mediated – pollen widely distributed in air. Very common, can be debilitating |
| | Contact dermatitis:<br>Oral – swelling and inflammation of mouth | Dumb cane (*Dieffenbachia*) | Calcium oxalate crystals coated with inflammatory proteins |
| | Skin – pain and stinging sensation | Nettles (*Urtica*) | Fine tubes contain histamine, acetylcholine and serotonin |

## 13.6.1 Skin

One of the best protections for a plant is to make skin contact painful. This is done through either an allergic antibody-mediated response or through direct-acting chemicals. For an allergic-type response it is not the first contact that produces the reaction but rather the next contact. Poison ivy produces a class of chemicals called urushiol that cause a very variable allergic response in about 70% of people exposed. Although not a direct protection for the plant, pollen of ragweed, mugwort, or grasses cause an allergic response in many people.

*Dieffenbachia* or dumb cane, a common houseplant, produces a juice that is released when a stem is broken or chewed and causes a painful rapid swelling and inflammation of the tongue and mouth. The symptoms can take several days to resolve and are caused by oxalate crystals coated with an irritating protein. Stinging nettles (*Urtica*) release histamine, acetylcholine, and serotonin from fine tubes with bulbs at the end that break off in the skin causing an intense burning or stinging sensation.

## 13.6.2 Gastrointestinal system

For the plant, another good way to stop consumption by an animal is to affect the animal's gastrointestinal system. This approach is used by a number of plants, but the mechanism of action varies. The first approach is direct irritation of the stomach lining to induce nausea and vomiting. The induction of mild vomiting is useful in some situations. The "sacred bark" of the California buckthorn produces cascara that is used to induce mild vomiting (a purgative).

**Table 13.6 Gastrointestinal system**

| Organ system | Symptoms | Plant examples | Toxin/comment |
|---|---|---|---|
| Gastrointestinal | Direct stomach irritation – nausea, vomiting and diarrhea | California buckthorn (sacred bark), tung nut, horse chestnut, pokeweed | Emodin and esculine (toxins); oil from seeds, nuts; some medical uses Children are most often affected |
| | Antimitotic (stops cell division) – nausea, vomiting, confusion, delirium | Lily family, glory lily, crocus, may apple | Colchicine (gout treatment) |
| | Lectin toxicity – nausea, diarrhea, headache, confusion, dehydration, death | Wisteria, castor bean (*Ricinus communis*) | Lectins bind to cell surfaces Ricin – blocks protein synthesis, very toxic, 5 to 6 beans can kill a child |

Other approaches to induce gastrointestinal discomfort have far more serious toxic effects. The chemical colchicine stops cell division (an antimitotic), producing severe nausea, vomiting, and dehydration, which can lead to delirium, neuropathy, and kidney failure. On the other hand, colchicine is used in the treatment of gout and has been studied as an anticancer agent because it stops cell division. Most toxic of all are plants that produce lectins, and the most toxic of these is the chemical ricin produced by castor beans. Only 5 to 6 seeds are necessary to kill a small child. Fortunately, following oral consumption much of the ricin is destroyed in the stomach. Ricin is extremely effective at stopping protein synthesis, so much so that direct exposure to only 0.1 μg/kg can be fatal.

### 13.6.3 Cardiovascular system

The medically important, cardiovascular drug digitalis was derived from foxglove (*Digitalis purpurea*). At medically useful doses, digitalis slows and stabilizes the heart rate, but at high dose it produces an irregular heart rate and decreased blood pressure. The Greeks first reported "mad honey poisoning" almost 2500 years ago, and honey poisoning still affects people around the world. The cardiovascular effects are caused by grayanotoxin, which is produced in the leaves and nectar of rhododendrons. The bees concentrate the toxin in the honey. Goats and sheep are also affected when they consume the leaves of rhododendron or some lily plants. The cardiovascular effects of consuming mistletoe contributed to some thinking it had either holy or demonic powers. The first more scientific observations on the cardiovascular effects of consuming mistletoe berries were in 1597.

### 13.6.4 Nervous system

There are many plants that produce a wide variety of substances that can affect the nervous system. We have exploited the nervous system effects of plants for thousands

**Table 13.7 Cardiovascular system**

| Organ system | Symptoms | Plant examples | Toxin/comment |
|---|---|---|---|
| Cardiovascular | Digitalis-like glycosides – cardiac arrhythmias | Foxglove (*Digitalis purpurea*), squill, lily-of-the-valley | Contain glycosides that are similar to digitalis – scillaren, convallatoxin |
| | Heart nerves – decreased heart rate and blood pressure, general weakness | Lily, hellebore, death camas, heath family, monkshood, rhododendron | Alkaloids, aconitum, grayanotoxin (concentrated in honey) |
| | Blood vessel constriction (vasoconstriction) | Mistletoe (berries contain toxin) | Holy or demonic – effects on heart first described in 1597. Toxin is called phoratoxin. |

of years and we continue to derive great value from some plants. In 399 BC. Socrates died from a dose of the Greek state poison extracted from hemlock. An interesting story possibly about a poison found in hemlock is found in the Bible, Book of Numbers, 11:31–33. Hungry Israelites died after eating quail blown in from the sea. Some have speculated that the quail had consumed seeds from hemlock that contained coniine. The quail are not affected by coniine, but it is stored in their tissue making them deadly for humans to eat.

The production and sale of coffee is a large international business solely designed to satisfy the demand for caffeine, the most widely consumed stimulant in the world. Mushrooms present another interesting challenge. Every year people are sickened and even die from eating poison mushrooms, while others consume them for their hallucinogenic effects.

In Table 13.8 is a brief look at some of the plants that produce neuroactive substances.

### 13.6.5 Liver

Fungi produce two of the most potent toxins affecting the liver. The "death cap" and "death angel" mushrooms from the *Amanita* family kill several people every year when they mistakenly consume these mushrooms (see case study example). There are also a number of fungi and molds that grow on nuts or grain. High humidity and poor storage conditions encourage the growth of a fungus on nuts that produces aflatoxin, a very potent toxin that causes liver cancer. People with prior liver disease such as hepatitis are particularly susceptible.

### 13.6.6 Reproductive effects

Reproductive and developmental toxins are primarily a concern for livestock. A high rate of fetal malformations in sheep offspring occurs following grazing on *Veratrum californicum* growing in the mountains of North America. Plants that induce abortion, such as bitter melon seeds, have a long history of use of in humans.

**Table 13.8 Nervous system**

| Organ system | Symptoms | Plant examples | Toxin/comment |
|---|---|---|---|
| Nervous system | Seizures | Water hemlock, (parsley family), mint family | Cicutoxin – effects potassium channels. Monoterpenes in mint oils |
| | Stimulation – excitatory amino acids – headache, confusion, hallucinations | Red alga (red tide), Green alga Mushrooms – *Amanita* family (fly agaric), flat pea (*Lathyrus*) | Kainic acid, domoic acid – concentrated in shellfish, Ibotenic acid, muscarinic acid, (hallucinations) Latthyrism – motor neuron degeneration |
| | Aberrant behavior – very excitable, muscle weakness, death | Locoweed – Australian and Western US plant | Swainsonine toxin – liver enzyme inhibitor – well known to affect cattle |
| | Stimulation | Coffee bean, tea, cola nut | Caffeine, most widely consumed stimulant in the world |
| | Neurotoxic – death | Poison hemlock (*Conium maculatum*) | Coniine – neurotoxic alkaloid – poison used by Socrates |
| | Paralysis – demyelination of peripheral nerves | Buckthorn, coyotillo, tullidora (US, Mexico) | Anthracenones – attack the myelin that surrounds the peripheral nerves |
| | Atropine-like effects – dry mouth, dilated pupils, confusion, hallucinations, memory lose | *Solanaceae* family – jimsonweed, henbane, deadly nightshade (*Atropa belladonna*), angles trumpet (atropine and scopolamine) | Clinical effects of many of the plants recognized since ancient times. Deaths are rare but children vulnerable. Hallucinations from muscarine and psilocybin |
| | Neuromuscular – mild stimulation to muscle paralysis, respiratory failure (curare), death | Tobacco – South American – *Strychnos* family (curare) Blue green alga (anatonin A) | Nicotine – blocks acetylcholine receptors Curare – used as a hunting poison, very potent receptor blocker |

## 13.7 Regulatory standards

Government regulatory agencies monitor some toxins as potential food contaminants. For example, agencies routinely monitor shellfish for several toxins and when necessary issue restrictions on harvesting. Many of the naturally occurring toxins are unregulated and the consumer must be aware of the potential hazards. It is really

**Table 13.9 Liver**

| Organ system | Symptoms | Plant examples | Toxin/comment |
|---|---|---|---|
| Liver | "Hepatitis" and cirrhosis of liver – from contaminated grain | Ragwort or groundsel | Pyrrolizidine alkaloids – attack liver vessels – affects humans and cattle, but some species resistant |
| | Liver failure and death | Mushrooms – "Death cap" (*Amanita phalloides*) | Amatoxin and phalloidin affect RNA and protein synthesis |
| | Liver cancer | Fungus that grows on peanuts, walnuts, etc. | Aflatoxins – produced by fungus in poorly stored grain |

**Table 13.10 Reproductive effects**

| Organ system | Symptoms | Plant examples | Toxin/comment |
|---|---|---|---|
| Reproductive effects | Teratogen – malformations in offspring (sheep) | *Veratrum californicum* – native to North America | Veratrum – blocks cholesterol synthesis – seen in offspring of mountain sheep |
| | Abortifacients – cause fetal abortions | Legumes (*Astrogalus*) Bitter melon seeds (*Momordica*) | Swainsonine toxin – stops cell division Lectins – halt protein synthesis – used by humans |

up to you, for example, to know what mushroom you consuming if you don't buy it at a store.

Note that some governments regulate noxious weeds, including some poisonous plants, but others are sold at garden stores.

## 13.8 Recommendation and conclusions

Children, because of their small size, are often the most susceptible to many of the naturally occurring toxins, just as they are to other toxicants. The caffeine from a can of cola will have a much bigger effect on a small child than it will on an adult. Health status and age, both young and old, also influence the response. Aflatoxin from contaminated nuts has a greater likelihood of causing cancer in someone with a liver disease such as hepatitis. It is important to develop a knowledge of which plants and animals can be dangerous and learn how to avoid dangerous contact with them.

## 13.9 More information and references

### 13.9.1 Slide presentation

- A Small Dose of Animal and Plant Toxins presentation material. Online. Available HTTP: <http://www.crcpress.com/e_products/> and follow the links to downloads and then the catalog number TF1691.
  Web site contains presentation material related to the health effects of animal and plant toxins.

### 13.9.2 European, Asian, and international agencies

- Society For The Study Of Amphibians And Reptiles (SSAR). Online. Available HTTP: <http://www.ku.edu/~ssar/> (accessed: 9 April 2003).
  SSAR – a not-for-profit organization established to advance research, conservation, and education concerning amphibians and reptiles.

### 13.9.3 North American agencies

- Health Canada – Natural Health Products Directorate. Online. Available HTTP: <http://www.hc-sc.gc.ca/hpfb-dgpsa/nhpd-dpsn/index_e.html> (accessed: 9 April 2003).
  Natural Health Products Directorate works to "ensure that all Canadians have ready access to natural health products that are safe, effective, and of high quality, while respecting freedom of choice and philosophical and cultural diversity".
- US Food and Drug Administration Center for Food Safety and Applied Nutrition. Online. Available HTTP: <http://www.cfsan.fda.gov/seafood1.html> (accessed: 9 April 2003).
  Site has information on seafood health and safety issues.
- Northwest Fisheries Science Center's (NWFSC) Marine Biotoxin Program. Online. Available HTTP: <http://www.nwfsc.noaa.gov/hab/index.htm> (accessed: 9 April 2003).
  NWFSC Marine Biotoxin Program, part of the US National Oceanic and Atmospheric Administration, "provides information and services to the public, state agencies, tribes, university, and others in the Eastern Pacific region".
- US Food & Drug Administration Center for Food Safety & Applied Nutrition Foodborne Pathogenic Microorganisms and Natural Toxins Handbook – The "Bad Bug Book". Online. Available HTTP: <http://www.cfsan.fda.gov/~mow/intro.html> (accessed: 9 April 2003).
  The "Bad Bug Book" contains extensive information on natural toxins either on the web or the book can be downloaded.

### 13.9.4 Non-government organizations

- Natural Toxins Research Center (NTRC) – Texas A&M University System. Online. Available HTTP: <http://ntri.tamuk.edu/> (accessed: 9 April 2003).

NTRC provides global research, training, and resources that will lead to the discovery of medically important toxins found in snake venoms.

- Cornell University Poisonous Plants Informational Database. Online. Available HTTP: <http://www.ansci.cornell.edu/plants/index.html> (accessed: 9 April 2003).
  This "includes plant images, pictures of affected animals and presentations concerning the botany, chemistry, toxicology, diagnosis and prevention of poisoning of animals by plants and other natural flora (fungi, etc.)".

- Alternative Medicine Foundation, Inc, HerbMed®. Online. Available HTTP: <http://www.herbmed.org/> (accessed: 9 April 2003).
  "HerbMed® – an interactive, electronic herbal database – provides hyperlinked access to the scientific data underlying the use of herbs for health. It is an evidence-based information resource for professionals, researchers, and general public."

- American Association of Poison Control Centers (AAPCC). Online. Available HTTP: <http://www.aapcc.org/> (accessed: 9 April 2003).
  The AAPCC is a United States based organization of poison centers and interested individuals that coordinates information on common poisons.

- The Vaults of Erowid. Online. Available HTTP: <http://www.erowid.org/index.shtml> (accessed: 9 April 2003).
  The Vaults of Erowid web site contains information on a wide variety of natural plants and chemicals.

### 13.9.5 References

- *Handbook of Clinical Toxicology of Animal Venoms and Poisons* by J. Meier and J. White (eds), CRC Press, Boca Raton, 752 pp. 1995.
- MMWR (1995) Jimson weed poisoning – Texas, New York, and California, 1994. Vol 44(3), 41–44. Online. Available HTTP: <http://www.cdc.gov/mmwr/preview/mmwrhtml/00035694.htm> (accessed: 5 July 2003).
- MMWR (1997) *Amanita phalloides* mushroom poisoning – Northern California, Vol 46(22), 489–491. Online. Available HTTP: <http://www.cdc.gov/mmwr/preview/mmwrhtml/00047808.htm> (accessed: 5 July 2003).
- MMWR (2002) Neurologic illness associated with eating Florida pufferfish, Vol 51(15), 321–323. Online. Available HTTP: <http://www.cdc.gov/mmwr/preview/mmwrhtml/mm5115a1.htm> (accessed: 5 July 2003).

# Chapter 14

## Persistent environmental contaminants

## Contents

- Dossier
- Case study
- Introduction and history
- Health effects
- Reducing exposure
- More information and references

### 14.1 Dossier

**Name:** persistent environmental contaminants (have various names depending on agency – i.e. US EPA persistent bioaccumulative and toxic (PBT) or United Nations persistent organic pollutant (POP)

**Use:** varies, often restricted or banned (but still present in the environment)

**Source:** industry, waste sites, food chain, and environment

**Recommended daily intake:** none (not essential)

**Absorption:** varies

**Sensitive individuals:** fetus, children

**Toxicity/symptoms:** range of toxic effects, developmental, learning and memory, cancer, etc.

**Regulatory facts:** various local, national, and international agencies working to eliminate or greatly reduce

**General facts:** long history of use, bioaccumulate

**Environmental:** global environmental contaminants

**Recommendations:** avoid, reduce use

## 14.2 Case study

From Advertisement for ORTHO Lindane – 1953

Check These ORTHO Lindane Advantages:
High Safety Factor – Authorities have approved Lindane for lice and mange control on dairy cattle. Shows no contamination in milk when properly applied. . . . Even used by dermatologists for human itch, lice and scabies. Not cumulative and practically odorless. Any taken in by a warm-blooded animal is eliminated.
  George S. Langford (ed.) *Entoma – A Directory of Insect and Plant Control*,
      10th edn, 1953–1954, Entomological Society of America, p. 165.

### 14.2.1 Lindane dumping site

Lindane (gamma-hexachlorocyclohexane) is one of the last of the old style organochlorine pesticides still in use. Use of organochlorines such as DDT, aldrin, dieldrin, heptachlor, and toxaphene is restricted or banned in many countries because of their persistence in the environment, bioaccumulation, and toxicity. Lindane was first isolated in 1825 along with other similar compounds, but its deadly effects on insects were not recognized until the 1940s.

Lindane was widely used because it killed a broad range of insects from fleas and ticks to worms that damaged crops. For a time it was even used to kill rodents. Lindane attacks the nervous system causing trembling, loss of coordination, paralysis, and ultimately death. Lindane was often applied as a spray on crops, where it would be either ingested or inhaled. Initially its environmental persistence was considered an asset, but eventually that was seen as a liability and led to restrictions in it use. Lindane is stable in water and has an average half-life of 15 months in soil. It is also highly toxic to fish; trout are affected at levels as low as 1.7 µg of lindane per liter of water. The US EPA restricted its use in 1983, as have most European countries. However, it continues to be used to treat seeds and is used in products to control head lice. In the US over 200,000 pounds are used each year to treat seeds prior to planting.

The US EPA set a drinking water limit of 0.2 parts per billion (ppb) of lindane. Industrial dumping sites such as the one in Allegheny County, Pennsylvania contain an estimated 400 tons of lindane waste and other waste dumped over a 50-year period on 30 acres of land. The runoffs from this site as well as others have the potential to contaminate drinking water with lindane. Lindane is regularly detected in surface water in the United States (see US Geological Survey monitoring studies).

## 14.3 Introduction and history

During the 1950s and 1960s there was an enormous increase in the use of chemicals in agriculture, industrial manufacturing, and around the home. We powdered our bodies with DDT to remove lice and spread DDT far and wide to control mosquitoes. We used other pesticides to kill insects and controlled weeds to improve crop yields. Lead was added to gasoline to make cars run better and added to house paint to make it last longer. At the same time we took advantage of the more sinister qualities of lead when we combined it with arsenic to spray on fruit trees to control pests. Pulp and paper mills used mercury to control fungi and molds to ensure that our paper remained white. Seeds were coated with mercury to stop soil fungi. Thermometers, thermostats, and switches brought mercury into everyone's home and school. Many will remember playing with a small ball of liquid silver mercury. Expansion of the electrical power system required chemicals that could withstand heat. For this purpose PCBs seemed to be the answer. All these chemicals appeared to be safe. A small dose did not seem harmful.

During the 1970s we began to appreciate that a small dose can harm sensitive individuals. Thirty years ago, in *Silent Spring*, Rachel Carson sounded one of the first alarms about the effects of environmental contaminants. Evidence accumulated that a pesticide like DDT can cause very unexpected effects. The first and most obvious was the thinning of bird eggshells, causing a sharp decline in predator bird populations. Predatory birds are at the top of the food chain, where they accumulate and concentrate DDT. Next we became aware of the potential of low-level exposures to these agents to cause diseases like cancer that appears only after many years. Humans at the top of the food chain accumulate DDT in fat. Fat is mobilized during lactation, and breast-feeding mothers pass the DDT to their infants. Small infants actually receives a large dose because of their low weight. We also learned that mercury and lead cause developmental effects, harming the developing nervous system for a lifetime.

It turns out that most of these compounds have similar characteristics that contribute to their toxicity to both humans and other species of plants and animals. First, the compounds are environmentally persistent. Many of the early pesticides, and certainly the metals, do not break down in the environment or do so only very slowly. If persistent chemicals are released continually to the environment, the levels tend to rise ever higher. This means they are available to cause harm to other organisms, often not even the target of the pesticide. Second, the early pesticides were broad acting and toxic to many species, not just the target species. These poisons often killed beneficial insects or plants. Third, many of these compounds would bio-accumulate or concentrate in species as they moved up the food chain. The chlorinated pesticides accumulate in the fat of animals. Animals that consumed other animals accumulated more and more of these pesticides. Most species could not metabolize or break down the compounds. Lead accumulates in bone and methyl mercury in muscle. And finally, because of their persistence in the environment and accumulation in various species, the persistent toxicants spread around the world even to places that never used them. Animals at the top of the food chain, such as polar bears and beluga whales, routinely have fat PCB levels greater that 6 ppm.

To address the public and environmental health concerns caused by these and other compounds, government agencies have initiated various programs and regulations to control or restrict the use of the offending compounds. Laws were passed to ensure increasing testing of compounds before widespread use, although this was not entirely effective. Researchers worked to develop new pesticides and other agents that were more specific in their toxicity and much less persistent. The use of many of the persistent chemical pesticides was restricted or even banned in some places. Individual countries are responsible for regulations, so there are some countries that still use pesticides banned in other countries.

Lists of persistent chemical pollutants are created to help prioritize efforts to reduce exposure. The United Nations Environment Programme (UNEP) created a list called persistent organic pollutants (POPs) that focuses on "chemical substances that persist in the environment, bioaccumulate through the food web, and pose a risk of causing adverse effects to human health and the environment". The UNEP also created a list of persistent toxic substances. The US EPA created a list of agents called persistent bioaccumulative and toxic (PBT) substances. Both these lists included organic chemicals and metals. Regional groups are also beginning to create lists of persistent chemical pollutants to emphasize and prioritize local issues. For example, Washington State Department of Ecology, in the United States, has created a list of persistent, bioaccumulative toxins (PBTs) to be phased out in the state. It is instructive to look at the overlap of these lists. The table below compares the lists of persistent chemical pollutants from these agencies. Overall there is considerable agreement as to what chemicals are considered a priority. It is also obvious that pesticides are a major class of persistent chemicals (Table 14.1).

## 14.4 Health effects

Table 14.2 provides a very brief description of the chemicals and associated toxicity. Additional information on individual agents can be found elsewhere in this book as well as many other sources.

## 14.5 Reducing exposure

Exposure depends on region of the world, diet, housing, occupation, and other factors. For example, methyl mercury bioaccumulates in certain fish and is particularly toxic to the developing fetus. Many government agencies advise that women of childbearing age or children reduce their consumption of certain species of fish know to bioaccumulate methyl mercury. Reducing exposure to persistent chemical pollutants is difficult because they are so pervasive and continue to build up over time. While individuals can sometimes reduce exposure to particular PBTs, such as mercury, by regulating their diet, in general government agencies have found that the most effective way of reducing exposure is by phasing out the uses of the products or processes that create these chemicals.

Many of the chemicals identified as persistent chemical pollutants are pesticides. Integrated pest management (IPM, see below for definition) is an approach to pest control that can significantly reduce pesticide use while still providing adequate or even improved results. IPM programs are used in agriculture, landscaping, and indoor pest control. Typically, IPM programs maximize prevention of pest problems through non-chemical methods, and chemicals, when used, are selected for minimum risk to non-targeted species.

> Integrated Pest Management (IPM) is a sustainable approach to managing pests by combining biological, cultural, physical and chemical tools in a way that minimizes economic, health and environmental risks.
>
> Anonymous, *Integrated Pest Management Practices on 1991 Fruits and Nuts, RTD Updates: Pest Management*, 1994, USDA-ERS, 8 pp.

**Table 14.1 Classification of persistent chemicals**

| Chemical | EPA | WA State | UN (POPs) | UN (PTSs) | Class |
|---|---|---|---|---|---|
| Aldrin/dieldrin | X | X | X | X | Pesticide |
| Benzo(a)pyrene | X | X | | | A PAH (see below) |
| Cadmium | | x | | | Metal |
| Chlordane | X | X | X | X | Pesticide |
| DDT, DDD, DDE | X | X | X | X | Pesticide |
| Dicofol | | X | | | Pesticide |
| Dioxins (TCDD) and furans | X | X | X | | Combustion byproducts |
| Endrin | | | X | X | Pesticide |
| Endosulfan | | X | | | Pesticide |
| Hexachlorobenzene | X | X | X | X | Pesticide |
| Heptachlor | | X | | X | Pesticide |
| alkyl-Lead | X | X | X | | Metal |
| Lindane | | X | | X | Pesticide |
| Mercury | X | X | | X | Metal |
| Methoxychlor | | X | | | Pesticide |
| Mirex | X | | X | X | Pesticide |
| Octachlorostyrene | X | | | | Byproduct |
| Polychlorinated biophenyls (PCBs) | X | X | X | X | Heat resistant |
| Pendimethalin | | X | | | Pesticide |
| Pentabromo diphenyl ether | | X | | | Former flame retardant |
| Pentachloronitrobenzene | | X | | | Pesticide |
| Polybrominated hydrocarbons | | | | X | Contaminate |
| Polycyclic aromatic hydrocarbons (PAHs) | | X | | X | Combustion byproducts |
| 1,2,4,5-Tetrachlorobenzene | | X | | | Pesticide |
| Tin (organotins) | | | | X | Metal |
| Toxaphene | X | X | X | X | Pesticide |
| Trifluralin | | X | | | Pesticide |

**Table 14.2 Chemicals and toxicity**

| Chemical | Comment |
| --- | --- |
| Aldrin/dieldrin | Pesticide – organochlorine – bioaccumulates – used to control mosquitoes and termites<br>Importation and manufacture prohibited in the US in 1987 |
| Benzo(a)pyrene | A PAH (see below under PAH) |
| Cadmium | Metal – naturally occurring – used in steel and plastics, batteries, cigarette smoke – lung carcinogen |
| Chlordane | Pesticide – organochlorine – bioaccumulates – used to control mosquitoes and termites<br>Importation and manufacture prohibited in the US, use banned in 1988 |
| DDT, DDD, DDE | Pesticide – organochlorine – bioaccumulates – used to control mosquitoes<br>Importation and manufacture prohibited in the US in 1972. Affects wildlife – found in breast milk and fat |
| Dicofol | Pesticide – organochlorine – bioaccumulates – insecticide on fruits – analog of DDT – degrades but very toxic to aquatic wildlife including fish |
| Dioxins (TCDD) and furans | Byproduct of combustion – bioaccumulates – municipal and medical waste incinerators – human carcinogen |
| Endrin | Pesticide – organochlorine – bioaccumulates – insecticide used on many crops – most use canceled in 1980 |
| Endosulfan | Pesticide – organochlorine – bioaccumulates – currently used as an insecticide |
| Heptachlor epoxide | Pesticide – organochlorine – bioaccumulates – heptachlor epoxide is a breakdown product of heptachlor, an insecticide from 1953 to 1974 in US on a wide range of insects.<br>Most use canceled in 1974 and importation and manufacture prohibited in the US, use banned in 1988 |
| Hexachlorobenzene | Pesticide – organochlorine – bioaccumulates – fungicide used in seeds<br>Most use ended in 1965 but is a byproduct in solvent manufacture |
| Lead | Metal – widely distributed in environment when used as a gasoline additive and in paint.<br>Now banned from use in gasoline and paint. Potent child neurotoxicant |
| Lindane | Pesticide – organochlorine – bioaccumulates – insecticide widely used prior to 1983<br>Regulated as drinking water contaminant by US EPA |
| Mercury | Metal – persistent – bioaccumulates – contaminates many species of fish. Widely used in industrial processes. Causes developmental neurotoxicity – children most susceptible |
| Methoxychlor | Pesticide – organochlorine – bioaccumulates – used as a replacement for DDT<br>In the US, 3.7 million pounds manufactured in 1978. Use has declined significantly – regulated has a water contaminant |

## Table 14.2 (cont'd)

| Chemical | Comment |
|---|---|
| Mirex | Pesticide – organochlorine – bioaccumulates – extensively used in US from 1962–1978 to control fire ants<br>All use canceled in US in 1978 |
| Octachlorostyrene | Byproduct of electrolytic production of magnesium. Listed by US EPA as persistent and bioaccumulative |
| Pendimethalin | Pesticide – herbicide used to control grasses and broadleaf weeds in crop fields and turf |
| Pentabromo diphenyl ether | Formerly used as flame retardant |
| Pentachlorobenzene | Pesticide – fungicide used for treatment of seeds and soil |
| Polybrominated hydrocarbons | Used in the manufacture of plastic products. Bioaccumulate and are highly persistent in the environment |
| Polychlorinated biophenyls (PCBs) | Heat and fire resistant – extensively used from 1929 and 1977 in electrical transformers<br>All manufacture banned – extensively regulated – very widespread global contaminant |
| Polycyclic aromatic hydrocarbons (PAHs) | Combustion byproducts – class of 100 chemicals – combustion byproducts from oil to tobacco. Some of the first known carcinogens |
| 1,2,4,5-Tetrachlorobenzene | Pesticide – insecticide and intermediate in herbicide production – related to dioxin (TCDD) |
| Tin (organotins) | Organotins are used in a number of consumer products including paint as a pesticide. Bioaccumulate and persistent, affects nervous system |
| Toxaphene | Pesticide – organochlorine – bioaccumulates – extensively used on US cotton crops from 1947 to 1980<br>Manufacture and use prohibited in the US |
| Trifluralin | Pesticide – herbicide used to control grasses and broadleaf weeds in crop fields and landscapes |

## 14.6 More information and references

### 14.6.1 Slide presentation

- A Small Dose of Persistent Environmental Contaminants presentation material. Online. Available HTTP: <http://www.crcpress.com/e_products/> and follow the links to downloads and then the catalog number TF1691. Web site contains presentation material related to this book for each chapter.

### 14.6.2 European, Asian, and international agencies

■ United Nations Environment Programme (UNEP) – Persistent Organic Pollutants (POP). Online. Available HTTP: <http://irptc.unep.ch/pops/default.html> (accessed: 9 April 2003).
Information on international efforts to reduce persistent pollutants.

### 14.6.3 North American agencies

■ Health Canada – Polychlorinated Biphenyls (PCBs). Online. Available HTTP: <http://www.hc-sc.gc.ca/english/iyh/environment/pcb.html> (accessed: 9 April 2003).
Health Canada provides information on the health effects and environmental distribution of PCBs.
■ US Environmental Protection Agency – Persistent Bioaccumulative and Toxic (PBT) Chemical Program. Online. Available HTTP: <http://www.epa.gov/opptintr/pbt/> (accessed: 9 April 2003).
Information of the efforts of US EPA to reduce PBT chemicals.
■ US Geological Survey. Online. Available HTTP: <http://www.usgs.gov/> (accessed: 9 April 2003).
This site contains information on the use of pesticides across the US, both as contaminants and crop use.
■ Washington State Department of Ecology – Persistent, Bioaccumulative Toxins. Online. Available HTTP: <http://www.ecy.wa.gov/programs/eap/pbt/pbtfaq.html> (accessed: 9 April 2003).
Information on this site states approach to persistent, bioaccumulative toxins.
■ US Department of Agriculture – Integrated Pest Management (IPM). Online. Available HTTP: <http://www.reeusda.gov/ipm/> (accessed: 9 April 2003).
Site provides information and other links on IPM.

### 14.6.4 Non-government organizations

■ Pesticide Action Network UK. Online. Available HTTP: <http://www.pan-uk.org/banlindane/> (accessed: 9 April 2003).
Site has information on the history and use of lindane and information on efforts to ban the use of lindane in Europe.
■ Pesticide Action Network North America (PANNA). Online. Available HTTP: <http://www.panna.org> (accessed: 9 April 2003).
"PANNA works to replace pesticide use with ecologically sound and socially just alternatives."
■ Washington Toxics Coalition (WTC). Online. Available HTTP: <www.watoxics.org> (accessed: 9 April 2003).
WTC provides information on model pesticide-policies, alternatives to home pesticides, information on persistent chemical pollutants, and much more.
■ Beyond Pesticides. Online. Available HTTP: <http://www.beyondpesticides.org/> (accessed: 9 April 2003).

"Beyond Pesticides is a national network committed to pesticide safety and the adoption of alternative pest management strategies which reduce or eliminate a dependency on toxic chemicals."

■  Northwest Coalition for Alternatives to Pesticides (NCAP). Online. Available HTTP: <http://www.pesticide.org/> (accessed: 9 April 2003).
"NCAP works to protect people and the environment by advancing healthy solutions to pest problems."

■  University of California Statewide Integrated Pest Management Program (UC IPM). Online. Available HTTP: <http://www.ipm.ucdavis.edu/> (accessed: 9 April 2003).
"UC – IPM develops and promotes the use of integrated, ecologically sound pest management programs in California."

■  Environmental Defense Fund – The Arctic at Risk: A Circumpolar Atlas of Environmental Concerns. Online. Available HTTP: <http://rainbow.ldgo. columbia.edu/edf/> (accessed: 9 April 2003).
Site has maps and information on contaminants in the arctic.

## 14.6.5 References

■  Atkin, J. and Klaus, M. Leisinger (eds). (2000) *Safe and effective use of crop protection products in developing countries*, CABI Publishing, CAB International, Wallingford, Oxon, UK, 163 pp.

■  Carson, R. (1994) *Silent Spring*. Houghton Mifflin, Boston, 368 pp.

■  Wargo, J. (1998) *Our children's toxic legacy: How science and law fail to protect us from pesticides*, 2nd edn, Yale University Press, 402 pp.

Part 2

# Targets of toxic agents

# Chapter 15

## Neurotoxicology

## Contents

- Introduction
- What is neurotoxicity?
- Case studies
- Biology of the nervous system
- What causes neurotoxicity?
- Who is vulnerable?
- Regulatory standards
- Recommendation and conclusions
- More information and references

## 15.1 Introduction

The human brain is the most complex structure known. It is only in the last few decades that we have begun to appreciate truly its flexibility, its complexity, and its vulnerability. The flexibility of the human nervous system is remarkable: when our ancient ancestors struggled for survival they were dependent on fire, hunting, and caves for shelter, while we rely on electricity, the supermarket, and central heating and cooling. For most, our ability to process complex information is far more important than our strength and reflexes. The brain's complexity is evident by the billons of cells that form more billions upon billions of connections, and all this takes place in a remarkably small confined space. In turn, these cells communicate using different chemicals called neurotransmitters. Neurotransmitters are frequently the target of drugs and chemicals that affect the nervous system. Prozac, a drug used to treat mild depression, affects the neurotransmitter serotonin. Lastly, the vulnerability of the nervous system to both transient effects and permanent damage from a wide variety of agents is increasingly evident. For thousands of years humans have searched out agents that affect the nervous system. Many people are regular users of alcohol or caffeine, as well as many other agents designed to affect the nervous system. Industrialization ushered in an era of rapid development of new chemicals with ever expanding use in our society, often accompanied by human exposure that we then learned, through sometimes tragic experience, can irreparably damage the nervous system. No one can reach his or her full genetic potential with a damaged nervous system. As a consequence, neurotoxicology developed in the 1970s to advance our understanding of the effects of chemicals on the nervous system.

> The upsurge of interest in recent years in academia, industry, and government on the effects of toxic chemicals on the nervous system has created a new discipline of neurotoxicology.
>
> Peter S. Spencer and Herbert H. Schaumberg, in *Experimental and Clinical Neurotoxicology*, 1980.

## 15.2 What is neurotoxicity?

**Neurotoxicity or a neurotoxic effect** – an adverse change in the chemistry, structure or function of the nervous system following exposure to a chemical or physical agent.

Voluntarily and involuntarily, we are exposed to a range of chemicals that affect the nervous system. We spend billions of dollars every year voluntarily purchasing chemicals such as caffeine, alcohol, and nicotine to influence our nervous system. Most stores and many industries are dependent on our desire to influence our nervous system. Many of us are familiar with the undesirable effects of too much caffeine or alcohol, which is a form of neurotoxicity. Fortunately, we quickly recover from the neurotoxic effects of caffeine or alcohol and from these experiences we learn to manage our consumption of these chemicals to minimize any undesirable effects and maximize the desirable effects. In this sense, many of us are experienced neurotoxicologists.

Voluntary consumption of chemicals (drugs) that our society has classified as illegal is also common. These drugs range from the active ingredient of the easily cultivated marijuana plant to chemicals produced in illicit laboratories. Billions of dollars are spent on the purchase of illegal drugs and in turn billions more are spent on trying to stop their manufacture and purchase. The direct and indirect costs to our society of the "war on drugs" are enormous.

A range of legal drugs is sold by the pharmaceutical industry to treat illnesses of the nervous system. Advances in our understanding of the structure and function of the nervous system has accelerated the development of chemicals for treating diseases such as Parkinson's syndrome, Alzheimer's disease, and mild depression. The treatment of mild depression with drugs like Prozac is a billion dollar industry. On the other hand, some drugs may produce undesirable nervous system side effects that can limit their utility in disease treatment. The anticancer drugs vincristine and cisplatin damage sensory nerves in the fingers and the anti-biotic gentomycin can affect hearing.

We are also involuntarily exposed to chemicals, compounds, or even physical agents that can damage the nervous system. The science of neurotoxicology has largely focused on understanding the adverse effects of agents on the nervous system. This research has shown that the nervous system, particularly the developing nervous system, is vulnerable to permanent damage by a number of agents. For ex-ample, even low levels of lead exposure will permanently damage the nervous system of young children, reducing their ability to learn and perform well in school, and ultimately affect their performance and quality of life as adults. Alcohol, while having a predictable effect on the pregnant mother, can be disastrous for the nervous system of the developing infant. Many workers are exposed to agents such as solvents or pesticides that can transiently affect the nervous system or even cause permanent damage. Physical agents such as noise and heat can also adversely affect the nervous system or degrade performance. Many people, including construc-tion workers who routinely use hearing protection devices, attest to the awareness that excessive exposure to loud noise will permanently damage hearing.

A more formal definition of neurotoxicity or a neurotoxic effect is an adverse change in the chemistry, structure, or function of the nervous system following exposure to a chemical or physical agent. An important part of this definition is that the effect may produce either structural change in the nervous system, such as gross cell loss, or function changes that may be related to subtle changes in nerve cell communication. Even minor changes in the structure or function of the nervous system may have profound consequences for neurological, behavioral, and related body functions. Often the very young and elderly are more susceptible to neurotoxic effects. Lead is a good example of a compound that at high levels of exposure can cause actual nerve cell damage but at low levels, particularly in children, can cause function losses such as decreased learning and memory.

Defining and testing for neurotoxicity is difficult because there is no one easy-to-define measure. Neurotoxicology effects can be divided into five areas (Table 15.1).

**Table 15.1 Neurological and behavioral effects of exposure to toxic substances**

| | |
|---|---|
| Motor effects | Convulsions, weakness, tremor, twitching, lack of coordination, unsteadiness, paralysis, reflex abnormalities, activity changes |
| Sensory effects | Equilibrium changes, vision disorders, pain disorders, tactile disorders, auditory disorders |
| Cognitive effects | Memory problems, confusion, speech impairment, learning impairment |
| Mood and personality effects | Sleep disturbances, excitability, depression, irritability, restlessness, nervousness, tension, delirium, hallucinations |
| General effects | Loss of appetite, depression of neuronal activity, narcosis stupor, fatigue, nerve damage |

Adapted from Anger (1986).

## 15.3 Case studies

### 15.3.1 Caffeine

Caffeine is the most widely consumed stimulant drug in the world. It occurs naturally in coffee, tea, and the cola nut and is added to many soft drinks. Many of us consume coffee and soft drinks because of the desirable stimulatory effects produced by caffeine; many of us have consumed too much caffeine and felt the consequences. The undesirable effects of caffeine, the agitation, the inability to concentrate, the mild tremors, and the general unpleasantness, are a form of neurotoxicity. Literally your brain, and more specifically, the adenosine receptors in your brain, has too much caffeine. These effects are a reversible form of neurotoxicity. Fortunately, we metabolize caffeine quickly and the undesirable effects end. By experience we have learned how to moderate our caffeine consumption to avoid the unpleasant side effects. A great deal of money is made from the neuroactive and physiological effects of caffeine. You can learn more about this fascinating drug in the chapter on caffeine.

### 15.3.2 Lead

The decision to use lead as a gasoline additive resulted in one of the greatest public health disasters of the twentieth century. Lead from the tail pipes of cars settled as dust over wide areas and was most prevalent in high traffic areas along city streets. Going from hand to mouth, the lead from cars and some additional lead from old lead-based paint was ingested by young children. In the 1970s and 1980s, researchers demonstrated that even low levels of lead exposure damaged the nervous system of children, confirming what the Greeks knew 2000 years ago: that "Lead makes the mind give way" (Dioscerides, second century BC). Exposure of the developing nervous system to lead causes irreversible harm, degrading the learning and memory capabilities of the child and resulting in a lifetime of deficit. While lead was banned from most paint and removed from gasoline, it still remains a threat to many children living in older homes with lead paint or near areas contaminated with lead. Lead is an example of a neurotoxic agent that causes permanent, irreversible damage to the developing nervous system, robbing a child of their genetic potential. You can learn more about the developmental effects of lead from the lead chapter.

### 15.3.3 Prozac (fluoxetine hydrochloride)

Prozac, produced by the pharmaceutical manufacturer Eli Lilly and Company, was first approved for the treatment of depression in Belgium in 1986. A year later, in 1987, it was approved for use in the United States. It is now approved for use in over 90 countries and used by more than 40 million people worldwide. Needless to say it is a very profitable drug.

Prozac is commonly prescribed for treatment of mild depression, which is not uncommon as we make our way through the dramas and disappointments of life. Prozac, similar to many neuroactive chemicals, has a remarkably specific effect on one neurotransmitter. Typically, a neurotransmitter is released from one cell to communicate across a very small gap to be picked up by a neuroreceptor on another cell. Once the neurotransmitter has performed its function of communicating with the other cell it is either degraded or taken back up by the releasing cell to be reused. Prozac functions by blocking this reuptake, thus leaving more neurotransmitter within the cell gap to continue stimulating the receiving cell. Prozac selectively inhibits the reuptake of the neurotransmitter serotonin. The increased availability of serotonin appears to reduce the symptoms of depression. A range of drugs, including the well-known hallucinogen LSD, acts through serotonin.

### 15.3.4 MPTP and Parkinson's disease

In the early 1980s, MPTP or 1-methyl-4-phenyl-1,2,3,6-tetrahydropyridine was accidentally produced as a contaminant of a new compound that clandestine chemists created in their search for a synthetic heroin. Tragically, drug users exposed to MPTP developed tremors and a lack of muscle control that was very similar to symptoms of Parkinson's disease. Parkinson's disease is usually a slow developing disease associated with the natural process of aging and the dying of cells in the brain. Further study revealed that MPTP attacked cells in a specific area of the brain that produce the neurotransmitter dopamine, the very same cells implicated in Parkinson's disease. This was the first time that a compound was clearly implicated in causing Parkinson's-like disease. Researchers immediately began searching for other compounds that might cause Parkinson's disease or interact with the aging processes to accelerate the onset of the disease. A number of studies have examined the association of exposure to some pesticides with an increase in Parkinson's disease. Researchers now use MPTP to develop animal models for finding new treatments for Parkinson's disease and to understand better the underlying progression of the disease.

## 15.4 Biology of the nervous system

### 15.4.1 Overview

The nervous system can be divided into the central nervous system (CNS), which includes the brain and spinal cord, and the peripheral nervous system (PNS), which carries information to and from the CNS. The PNS is the information highway while the CNS is the coordinating center. Sensory information such as touch or pain is transmitted to the CNS by the nerves of the PNS. If we touch something hot the CNS will then command, through the PNS, to move those muscles that will withdraw us from the pain. The CNS also communicates with a number of glands and organs through the PNS. In addition to the basic functions of keeping us alive, the brain is responsible for our thinking, reasoning, and emotions.

The brain is incredibly complex. It is estimated to contain between 10 billion and 100 billion cells that form approximately $10^{15}$ connections; a huge number when compared with the 42 million transistors on a state of the art microprocessor chip. The information processing capabilities of the brain are enormous. The nervous system starts developing early in gestation and continues to grow and change, particularly in the first few years of infancy and childhood. During development, the brain organizes into separate but interconnected areas that control different functions. For example, the area of the brain that processes visual information is located in the back of your head. During development, cells from the eyes must connect with cells of the optic nerve to move information to the visual processing center of the brain. This complex dance of one cell looking for a partner in another area of the brain is one reason the brain is so sensitive to disruption by a range of compounds.

The peripheral nerves are undergoing many similar challenges. Think of the longest nerves in your body that run from the bottom of your spinal cord to your toes. These very long cells must be able to connect, grow, and communicate with the right cells of the spinal cord, which in turns must communicate, with the cells of the brain.

### 15.4.2 Cells of the nervous system

The nervous system consists of cells, called neurons (Figure 15.1), which are responsible for the majority of information transfers in the central and peripheral nervous systems and supporting cells. In the PNS, the neurons can be very long. For example, consider the information that must be sent to and from your fingers or toes to either sense touch or pain or move the muscles. The neurons have a cell body and a long connecting structure called an axon. To increase the transmission speed along the axon, another cell, a Schwann cell, wraps the axon to provide a form of insulation to facilitate the movement of electrical signals. The Schwann cells literally wrap themselves around the long axon forming multiple layers similar to tree rings. As will be discussed below these cells are susceptible to damage because of the long axon and the energy requirements of the cell.

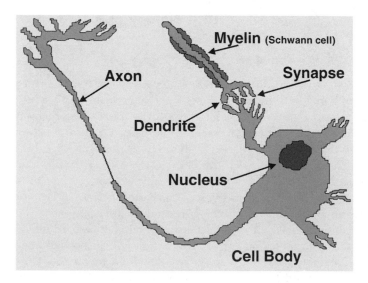

**Figure 15.1.** Neurons in the peripheral nervous system.

In the CNS, glial cells aid in the communication between the densely packed neurons of the CNS. These cells also play a big part in forming the blood–brain barrier. The blood–brain barrier keeps some classes of chemicals from entering the brain, which can make it very difficult to treat diseases of the brain. However, some chemicals, such as caffeine, readily enter the brain, as do many other neuroactive compounds. Compounds essential for function are actively transported across this barrier.

### 15.4.3 Transmission of information in the nervous system

Nerve cells communicate by the release of chemicals (neurotransmitters) into the space between the cells (Figure 15.2). The neurotransmitter is typically stored in a small packet (synaptic vesicle) and then released in response to a signal that is transmitted down the cell axon. In the example in Figure 15.2, dopamine, an important neurotransmitter involved in movement disorders related to Parkinson's disease, is released into the gap (synaptic cleft) and reacts with specific receptors on the adjacent cell. This in turn causes a reaction in the adjacent cell. Dopamine in the gap can either be broken down or taken back up into the cell that released it and repackaged for future use.

In Parkinson's disease the dopamine-releasing cells are damaged or die, thus reducing the release of dopamine. Loss of the dopamine neurotransmitter contributes to the movement disorders associated with Parkinson's disease. Typically, the loss of dopamine-producing cells in a very specific location in the brain does not become evident until old age, and for a long time Parkinson's disease was thought of as

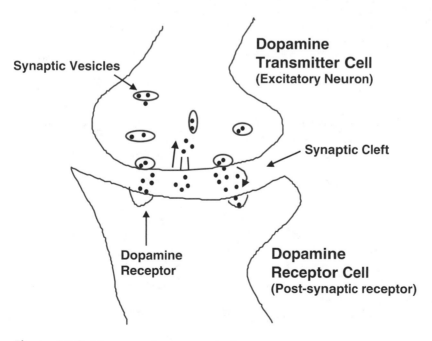

*Figure 15.2.* Nervous system communication.

strictly age related. In the 1970s this concept was changed when chemists produced a designer drug meant to mimic common narcotics that had an impurity that resulted in a Parkinson's-like syndrome in young people never thought to be susceptible to Parkinson's disease. A specific compound, MPTP, was found to cause the death of the dopamine-producing cells in the same area of the brain. While the consequence to the individuals was tragic, MPTP has proven to be a very important research tool for understanding this disease as well as developing new treatments.

## 15.5 What causes neurotoxicity?

There is no simple or correct way to examine the causes of neurotoxicity. I have divided them into three overlapping areas: neurotransmitter/receptor effects, which are often transient; damage to the peripheral nerves, which is often permanent; and damage to the developing nervous system, which is almost always permanent.

Nerve cells have unique structural and physiological features that often make them more susceptible to damage from chemical agents. Cells of the central nervous system have a high metabolic rate that makes them highly dependent on glucose and oxygen, much like computer chips need lots of electrical power. Anything that disrupts the flow of glucose or energy utilization within the cell causes a loss of function and potentially long-term damage. Nerve cells, unlike muscle cells, can only work for a very short time without oxygen. The most obvious indicator of this is that we quickly lose consciousness when our brain is deprived of well-oxygenated blood. Agents like carbon monoxide reduce the availability of oxygen to the brain resulting quickly in unconsciousness or even death. Cyanide, working by a very different mechanism, inhibits a cell's ability to utilize oxygen, which produces the same results. In the peripheral nervous system, the length of cells contributes to their increased susceptibility to damage from agents that disrupt the transfer of nutrients along the length of the cell. Acrylamide, for example, causes damage to the cell transport system, which results in paralysis that is first noticed in the legs.

In the majority of cases, the cells of the nervous system cannot divide and replace themselves, thus most damage is permanent. The developing nervous system exposed to lead will be damaged for a lifetime. However, peripheral nerves can grow, recovering some of the connections and functionality that results in some sensation and return of movement, usually most noticeable in the arms and legs.

### 15.5.1 Neurotransmitter/receptor effects

Many naturally occurring compounds and an increasing number of synthesized chemicals work by influencing the effectiveness of a specific neurotransmitter. Typically, neurotransmitters are released from one neuronal cell and are picked up by specific receptors in the adjacent cell, which causes the receiving cell to react. The receptor then releases the neurotransmitter into the gap between the cells. At this time the neurotransmitter must be removed either by being broken down by a specific enzyme or it can be taken back up by the releasing cell to be reused. A compound can influence a neurotransmitter and thus the response of the receiving cell in several ways:

### Table 15.2 Mechanism of action of neuroactive agents

| Compound | Neurotransmitter | Action |
|---|---|---|
| Caffeine | Blocks the adenosine receptor | Stimulant |
| Organophosphate insecticides | Increases the neurotransmitter acetylcholine by blocking its degradation | Stimulant |
| Nicotine | Mimics acetylcholine, thus looks like increased acetylcholine | Stimulant |
| Fluoxetine (Prozac) | Increases serotonin by blocking its reuptake into neuronal cells | Stimulant |
| LSD (lysergic acid diethylamide) | Mimics serotonin, thus stimulating receptor | Hallucination |
| THC-Delta 9-tetrahydro-cannabinol (cannabis) | Cannabinoid receptor | Relaxation, euphoria, and enhancement of senses, increase in appetite, sense of time |
| Cocaine | Blocks dopamine transporter, thus increasing dopaminergic stimnlation | Increases alertness and energy, euphoria, insomnia, restlessness, fear, paranoia, hallucinations. |
| Domoic acid (shellfish) | Glutamate, aspartate | Loss of memory |

(1) blocking the receptor so that the neurotransmitter cannot reach the receptor and thus the receiving cell is unable to respond
(2) mimicking the neurotransmitter so that the receiving cell responds even though there is no naturally occurring neurotransmitter
(3) blocking the degradation of the neurotransmitter, thus leaving the neurotransmitter to react with another receptor
(4) blocking the reuptake of the neurotransmitter into the release cell, which leaves the neurotransmitter free to react again with the receptor.

Table 15.2 provides just a few examples of different neuroactive agents and their mechanism of action. Caffeine, the most widely consumed stimulant drug in the world, works by affecting the adenosine receptor. Adenosine is a naturally occurring depressant, so caffeine works by blocking the depressive actions of adenosine, causing stimulation.

Agents acting through a specific neurotransmitter are often transient, and exposure must be repeated to continue the effect, witness our repeated need for caffeine every morning. This is not always the case. Very potent (poisonous) nerve gases permanently block the agent responsible for degrading acetylcholine, thus causing death because the nervous system cannot recover.

### 15.5.2 Damage to the peripheral nerves

The peripheral nerves of the body communicate sensation and deliver commands from the central nervous system to move muscles from our fingers to our toes – quite

**Table 15.3** Peripheral nervous system damage

| Name | Type | Example |
|---|---|---|
| Neuronopathy | Nerve cell death | MPTP, trimethyltin |
| Axonopathy | Degeneration of axon | Hexane, acrylamide |
| Myelinopathy | Damage to myelin (e.g. Schwann cells) | Lead, hexachlorophene |
| Transmission toxicity | Disruption of neurotransmission | Organophosphate pesticides, cocaine, DDT |

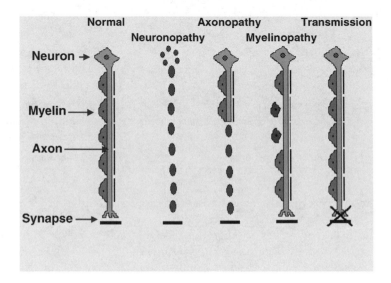

**Figure 15.3.** Peripheral nervous system damage.

a distance. Peripheral nerves are wrapped by a specialized cell to form an insulation (myelin) that aids the transmission of electrical signal up along the length of the nerve cell. Agents damage the peripheral nervous system either by killing the nerve cell (neuronopathy), attacking the axon (axonopathy), or by attacking the insulation that surrounds the cells (myelinopathy) (Table 15.3 and Figure 15.3). Interfering with the neurotransmitter is a form of transmission toxicity, which was discussed in more detail above.

### 15.3.3 Damage to the developing nervous system

The developing nervous system is more vulnerable to damage than the mature nervous system for a number of reasons. The blood–brain barrier of the central nervous system is not well developed in the very young, which allows toxic agents easy access to the nervous system. The nervous system develops through our gestation and continues changing well into our teens with cells multiplying, growing in size or length, migrating to a new location, or forming connections with other cells. During this period toxic agents may kill cells, interfere with their migration, or interfere with the cell-forming connections. Different areas of the nervous system develop at different times, so exposure to an agent such as alcohol during the fourth month of gestation will have different effects than exposure during the sixth month.

Damage to the brain can range from the severe and obvious to the very subtle and undetectable. Exposure to high levels of alcohol during gestation can cause obvious reductions in the ability of a child to perform well in school and even contribute to society. More difficult to assess is the damage caused by very low levels of exposure. Low levels of exposure to alcohol or lead during development may reduce a child's IQ only slightly, by a degree that is within the normal range of variation. These more subtle changes can only be examined by comparing large groups of people, some of whom are exposed to the agent and some who are not. Group-based studies such as these were the first to show that even low levels of lead exposure during development can cause subtle decreases in IQ, thus depriving an individual of the ability to reach their full genetic potential. Any one individual would not know if their intellectual capabilities had been reduced, but on a large scale these changes have serious implications for society. Additional information is available in the lead and alcohol chapters.

Another area of concern is exposure to fat-soluble compounds such as PCBs or chlorinated pesticides. All cells contain lipids or fat; the high number of densely packed cells of the brain means that the brain is just a big ball of fat. The brain is a great storage site for fat-soluble compounds that can cross the blood–brain barrier. An additional concern is that these compounds can be mobilized from the fat of women breastfeeding their infants, resulting in exposure to the infant and, given the size of the infant, this exposure translates into a large dose.

### 15.5.4 Diseases of the nervous system

Can toxic agents cause what have been classically defined as diseases of the nervous system, such as Parkinson's disease, Alzheimer's-type dementia, multiple sclerosis, or amyotrophic lateral sclerosis (ALS)? The discovery that the chemical MPTP can cause a syndrome very similar to Parkinson's disease really focused people's attention on the possibility that chemical agents may play a role in the onset of neurological disorders once exclusively thought to be associated with aging or just bad luck. MPTP selectively damaged the same neurons, in the same area of the brain, as those responsible for Parkinson's disease. Supporting the hypothesis that chemical agents may contribute to Parkinson's disease were data showing that the incidence of this disease had increased when compared with historical patterns, which correlated with the increased use and exposure to chemicals. Additional research showed that the active metabolite of MPTP, which was really responsible for damaging the neurons, was very similar to the chemical structure of some pesticides. This immediately raised the question: Could pesticide exposure increase the incidence of Parkinson's disease or cause the disease to occur at an earlier age? In fact, researchers did find some correlation with pesticide exposure in farm workers and the onset of Parkinson's disease.

Exposure to metals is associated with a number of neurological disorders, so it was reasonable to ask: Could exposure to metals contribute to age-related neurological disorders? Researchers found that brain cells of many Alzheimer's patients had elevated levels of aluminum, and kidney dialysis patients could suffer from a neurological disorder related to elevated exposure to aluminum, but much additional study has never found that aluminum exposure causes Alzheimer's disease. There is, however, some data supporting the possibility that exposure to mercury could result in accelerated age-related decline of cognitive function.

Neurological and psychiatric disorders such as depression, hyperactivity, and manic depression have driven many pharmaceutical companies and researchers to develop neuroactive drugs to treat these conditions. This is an active area of research that will accelerate as we gain more knowledge of the underlying mechanisms of the nervous system. Early drugs used to treat psychiatric disorders often had highly undesirable side effects that often limited their long-term use or required additional drugs to manage the complications. Newer drugs are more specific and have fewer side effects.

Table 15.4 lists a few examples of neurotoxicology caused by a variety of agents.

### Table 15.4 History of neurotoxicology

| Year(s) | Location | Substance | Comments |
|---|---|---|---|
| 400 BC to present | Worldwide | Lead | Hippocrates recognizes lead toxicity in the mining industry; lead used to sweeten Roman wine; modern – lead used in paint and as a gasoline additive; low level lead exposure shown to damage the nervous system of children |
| Ancient | Worldwide | Mercury | Mine workers poisoned; 1930s hat industry (the Mad Hatters); 1950s Japan, mercury in fish; 1970s mercury in seed grain; acceptance of mercury as a developmental neurotoxicant; released from coal-fired electrical plants; ongoing contamination of fish |
| 1930s | United States (southeast) | TOCP | Compound often added to lubricating oils contaminates "Ginger-Jake", an alcoholic beverage; more than 5000 paralyzed, 20 000 to 100 000 affected |
| 1930s | Europe | Apiol (w/TOCP) | Abortion-inducing drug containing TOCP causes 60 cases of neuropathy |
| 1932 | United States (California) | Thallium | Barley laced with thallium sulfate, used as a rodenticide, is stolen and used to make tortillas; 13 family members hospitalized with neurological symptoms; 6 deaths |
| 1937 | South Africa | TOCP | 60 South Africans develop paralysis after using contaminated cooking oil |
| 1950s | France | Organotin | Contamination of Stallinon with triethyltin results in more than 100 deaths |
| 1950s | Morocco | Manganese | 150 ore miners suffer chronic manganese intoxication involving severe neurobehavioral problems |

### Table 15.4 (cont'd)

| Year(s) | Location | Substance | Comments |
|---|---|---|---|
| 1950s–70s | United States | AETT | Component of fragrances found to be neurotoxic; withdrawn from market in 1978; human health effects unknown |
| 1956 | – | Endrin | 49 persons become ill after eating bakery foods prepared from flour contaminated with the insecticide endrin; convulsions resulted in some instances |
| 1956 | Turkey | HCB | Hexachlorobenzene, a seed grain fungicide, leads to poisoning of 3000 to 4000, 10 percent mortality rate |
| 1956–77 | Japan | Clioquinol | Drug used to treat travelers' diarrhea found to cause neuropathy; as many as 10 000 affected over two decades |
| 1959 | Morocco | TOCP | Cooking oil contaminated with lubricating oil affects some 10 000 individuals |
| 1968 | Japan | PCBs | Polychlorinated biphenyls leaked into rice oil, 1665 people affected |
| 1969 | Japan | n-Hexane | 93 cases of neuropathy occur following exposure to n-hexane, used to make vinyl sandals |
| 1971 | United States | Hexachlorophene | After years of bathing infants in 3 percent hexachlorophene, the disinfectant is found to be toxic to the nervous system and other systems |
| 1971 | Iraq | Mercury | Mercury used as fungicide to treat seed grain is used in bread; more than 5000 severe poisoning, 450 hospital deaths, effects on many infants exposed prenatally not documented |
| 1973 | United States (Ohio) | MnBK | Fabric production plant employees exposed to solvent; more than 80 workers suffer polyneuropathy, 180 have less severe effects |
| 1974–75 | United States (Hopewell, VA) | Chlordecone (Kepone) | Chemical plant employees exposed to insecticide; more than 20 suffer severe neurological problems, more than 40 have less severe problems |
| 1976 | United States (Texas) | Leptophos (Phosvel) | At least 9 employees suffer serious neurological problems following exposure to insecticide during manufacturing process |
| 1977 | United States (California) | Dichloropropene (Telone II) | 24 individuals hospitalized after exposure to pesticide Telone following traffic accident |
| 1979–80 | United States (Lancaster, TX) | BHMH (Lucel-7) | Seven employees at plastic bathtub manufacturing plant experience serious neurological problems following exposure to BHMH |
| 1980s | United States | MPTP | Impurity in synthesis of illicit drug found to cause symptoms identical to those of Parkinson's disease |

| Table 15.4 (cont'd) | | | |
|---|---|---|---|
| Year(s) | Location | Substance | Comments |
| 1981 | Spain | Toxic oil | 20,000 persons poisoned by toxic substance in oil, resulting in more than 500 deaths; many suffer severe neuropathy |
| 1985 | United States | Aldicarb | More than 1000 individuals in California and other Western States and British Columbia experience neuromuscular and cardiac problems following ingestion of melons contaminated with the pesticide aldicarb |
| 1987 | Canada | Domoic acid | Ingestion of mussels contaminated with domoic acid causes 129 illness and 2 deaths. Symptoms include memory loss, disorientation, and seizures |
| 1991 | United States | Domoic acid | Shellfish contaminated with domoic acid found in the Northwest |

Adapted from: Neurotoxicity: US Congress, office of Technology Assessment (1990).

| Table 15.5 Exposure to neurotoxic compounds | | |
|---|---|---|
| Home | (a) | children during development form maternal exposure |
| | (b) | children – lead in the home |
| | (c) | cleaning agents |
| | (d) | solvents |
| Workplace | (a) | solvents |
| | (b) | pesticides |
| Environment | (a) | lead |
| | (b) | mercury (in fish) |
| | (c) | pesticides |
| | (d) | persistent environmental pollutants |

## 15.6 Who is vulnerable?

Without a doubt the developing fetus and child are the most vulnerable to the effects of chemicals on the nervous system. As children they have no control over these exposures that can result in a lifetime of disability. The nervous system of adults is clearly affected by a range of chemicals, both those sought after and in our environment.

The home, workplace, and general environment each represent unique places of possible exposure to neuroactive agents (Table 15.5). The home contains a range of compounds that affect the nervous system: caffeine in coffee and tea, alcohol, medicines, pesticides, cleaning agents, paints, and solvents to name just a few. Compounds such a lead or pesticides can be carried into the home on shoes or bare feet. Working family members may bring agents such as lead home on clothing. Probably the greatest concern in the workplaces is solvent exposure from cleaning agents or chemical processes. Farmers and pesticide workers can also be exposed to compounds clearly designed to affect the nervous system. The outdoor environment can contain elevated levels of a number of persistent chemicals that can adversely affect the nervous system, such as lead, mercury, and chlorinated pesticides.

## 15.7 Regulatory standards

As our appreciation for the subtle neurological effects and long-term consequences of exposure to compounds has increased, there has been a gradual increase in the testing requirements for new compounds. Government agencies can now require additional testing for the neurotoxic effects of a compound. However, for many compounds we know very little about their potential to cause neurotoxicity or affect the developing nervous system. In the case of lead, there is no safety factor included in the levels of concern indicated by the Center for Disease Control, but rather, the standard was set based on a low level found in the general population as lead was removed from gasoline. In general, the government struggles to keep up with the ever-growing list of new chemicals and struggles to assess their potential to cause neurotoxic injury.

## 15.8 Recommendation and conclusions

Many of us regularly consume compounds that affect our nervous system and are well aware of chemicals that cause neurotoxicity, so the recommendation is simple – be aware. The developing nervous system is very sensitive to neurotoxicity and exposure to the wrong chemical at the wrong time can cause a lifetime of disability. From an ethical and social perspective this vulnerability of the developing nervous system represents unique challenges and responsibilities. Our expanding understanding of the nervous system combined with the knowledge of the subtle harm that can be done is one of the most important contributions of the toxicological sciences.

## 15.9 More information and references

### 15.9.1 Slide presentation

- A Small Dose of Neurotoxicology presentation material. Online. Available HTTP: <http://www.crcpress.com/e_products/> and follow the links to downloads and then the catalog number TF1691.
  Web site contains presentation material related to the neurotoxic effects of chemicals.

### 15.9.2 European, Asian, and international agencies

- Organization For Economic Co-Operation And Development (OECD) – Chemical Safety. Online. Available HTTP: <http://www.oecd.org/EN/home/

0,,EN-home-519-nodirectorate-no-no-no-12,00.html> (accessed: 10 April 2003).
This OECD site contains general information on chemical safety as well as specific testing guidelines for neurotoxic effects of chemicals.

■ International Neurotoxicology Association (INA). Online. Available HTTP: <http://www.neurotoxicology.org/> (accessed: 10 April 2003).
Site provides links to neurotoxicology testing guidelines and other information on neurotoxicology.

■ University of Stockholm, Department of Neurochemistry & Neurotoxicology. Online. Available HTTP: <http://www.neurochem.su.se/> (accessed: 10 April 2003).

■ International Brain Research Organization (IBRO). Online. Available HTTP: <http://www.ibro.org/index.htm> (accessed: 10 April 2003).
IBRO is a non-profit international organization for neuroscientists.

■ Universiteit Utrecht – Neurotoxicology and Immunotoxicology (RITOX). Online. Available HTTP: <http://www.ritox.vet.uu.nl/ntx.html> (accessed: 10 April 2003).
RITOX offers information and training in neurotoxicology.

### 15.9.3 North American agencies

■ US Food and Drug Administration (FDA) – Neurotoxicology Division Access: http://www.fda.gov/nctr/science/divisions/neurotox.htm> (accessed: 10 April 2003).
Information on FDA and neurotoxicology.

■ US Environmental Protection Agency (EPA) Neurotoxicology Division. Online. Available HTTP: <http://www.epa.gov/nheerl/ntd/> (accessed: 10 April 2003).
This EPA site provides information on neurotoxicology.

■ US National Institute of Health – National Institute of Neurological Disorders and Stroke (NINDS). Online. Available HTTP: <http://www.ninds.nih.gov/> (accessed: 10 April 2003).
NINDS is working to shape "the future of research and its relationship to brain diseases".

■ US National Research Council – Environmental Neurotoxicology. Online. Available HTTP: <http://www.nationalacademies.org/nrc/> (accessed: 10 April 2003).
Publication available on the web at this site.

### 15.9.4 Non-government organizations

■ Society for Neuroscience (SFN). Online. Available HTTP: <www.sfn.org/> (accessed: 10 April 2003).
"SFN is a nonprofit membership organization of basic scientists and physicians who study the brain and nervous system."

■ ALS Association (ALSA) (amyotrophic lateral sclerosis). Online. Available HTTP: <http://www.alsa.org/> (accessed: 10 April 2003).

The mission of The ALS Association is to find a cure for and improve living with ALS.

- Natural Resources Defense Council (NRDC). Online. Available HTTP: <http://www.nrdc.org/health/kids/cfqpa0599.asp> (accessed: 10 April 2003). NRDC site provides information on children's health and neurotoxicology.

### 15.9.5 References

- Anger, W. K. (1986). Workplace exposures, in *Neurobehavioral Toxicology*, Z. Annau (ed), Johns Hopkins University Press, Baltimore, MD, 443 pp.
- Chang, L. W. and Slikker, W., Jr. (eds). (1995). *Neurotoxicology: Approaches and Methods.* Academic Press San Diego, 851 pp.
- Spencer, P. S. and Schaumburg, H. H. (eds). (2000). *Experimental and Clinical Neurotoxicology*, 2nd edn Oxford University Press, 1152 pp.
- US Congress, Office of Technology Assessment, *Neurotoxicity: Identifying and Controlling Poisons of the Nervous System*, OTA-BA-436 (Washington, DC: US Government Printing Office, April 1990.), p. 47.

# Chapter 16

## Cancer and genetic toxicology

### Contents

- What is cancer?
- Case studies
- Biology of cancer and genetic toxicology
- What causes cancer?
- Who is vulnerable?
- Regulatory standards
- Recommendation and conclusions
- More information and references

## 16.1 What is cancer?

Cancer is an unwelcome, potentially life-threatening diagnosis that one-third of us will experience. The oldest descriptions of cancer date back to Egypt around 1600 BC. The so-called Edwin Smith Papyrus describes eight cases of what appears to be breast cancer. The tumors of the breast were treated by cauterization, with a tool called "the fire drill". Clearly there was a desire and need to treat this dreaded disease, but the conclusion was "There is no treatment". It is only in the last 100 years that we have developed more sophisticated tools to treat cancer.

We now know much more about cancer, its causes, and treatment. Technically cancer is the uncontrolled growth of cells that have damaged DNA expression. The cancerous cells repeatedly divide, displacing normal tissue. The cancer or neoplasm may be either benign or malignant. A benign cancer stays confined to the tissue of origin while malignant cancer can spread to other organs. The secondary growths or metastases are a serious complication to any treatment of the cancer cells. A tumor is any space-filling group of cells that may or may not be cancerous.

Benign growths or tumors are usually denoted by having the ending "-oma", for example, adenoma would be a benign growth of the adrenal cortex, a hormone-producing group of cells near the kidney. Malignant tumors are noted by adding "sarcoma" or "carcinoma". A malignancy of the adrenal cortex would be an adenocarcinoma. Bone cancer would be osteosarcoma.

Toxicology informs us about cancer on two accounts. First, toxicology research provided insight into the causes of cancer and likelihood of developing cancer. Second, many of the treatments for cancer have serious toxicological side effects. Cancer treatment must often balance the need to kill the cancerous cells while limiting the damage to the normal cells of the body.

Initially, our understanding of cancer was advanced entirely by humans, the ultimate experimental subject. The first occupational association with cancer was noted in 1700 with the observation that nuns had an elevated incidence of breast cancer. In 1775, the English physician and surgeon, Percivall Pott, made the very astute observation that exposure to soot might explain the high incidence of cancer of the scrotum in chimney sweeps (Table 16.1). This was the first indication that exposure to chemicals, in this case a complex mixture, could cause cancer. This new knowledge did not immediately translate into improved working conditions for chimney sweeps. Over 100 years later it was observed that cancer of the scrotum was rare in continental Europe but still high in England, possibly due to better hygiene practices in Europe. We still have not taken to heart the cancerous consequences of exposure to smoke and tar as ongoing consumption of tobacco products clearly shows.

The industrial revolution of the late nineteenth and early twentieth century brought clear confirmation that occupational exposure to chemicals could cause cancer. The first indication came from increases in skin and bladder cancers associated with cutting oils and dyes. In 1895 bladder cancer was associated with workers in the aniline dye industry. Further worker-based studies found that exposure to

**Table 16.1 Selected history of cancer**

| Year | Cancer type | Cause |
|------|-------------|-------|
| 1775 | Scrotal cancer | Soot |
| 1822 | Skin cancer | Arsenic |
| 1879 | Lung cancer | Uranium miners |
| 1895 | Bladder cancer | Aniline dye |
| 1902 | Skin cancer | X-rays |
| 1908 | Leukemia | Filterable agent |
| 1914 | Experimental induction of skin cancers (rabbit) | Coal Tar |
| 1928 | Experimental induction of skin cancers | UV Light |

specific chemicals could be responsible for the cancer. In 1915 Japanese researchers reported that they could induce skin tumors in animals by repeatedly applying a coal tar solution to the skin of rabbits. These early studies, subsequently repeated with mice, ushered in the scientific investigation of the chemical cause of cancer. These early animals studies initiated the systematic investigation of the adverse effects of chemicals, which in many ways laid the foundation for the toxicological sciences.

But chemicals are not the only cause of cancer. During this incredible period of time, researchers such as Marie Curie (1867–1934) were discovering radioactivity and in 1895 Wilhem Conrad Roentgen discovered X-rays. Marie Curie was ultimately awarded Nobel Prizes in both physics and chemistry, the only person ever so honored. One of her discoveries was radium in 1898. The green glow of radium fascinated people and many thought it was a cure for many diseases, including cancer. The carcinogenicity of radium became tragically apparent when young women developed bone cancer from painting watch dials with radium (for more details see the radiation chapter). The use of nuclear weapons by the US military and subsequent development of the defense and nuclear industries has made us all well aware of the consequence of radiation exposure. Naturally occurring background radiation combined with our many medical and industrial exposures to radiation is responsible for some cancers.

As our observational powers improved so did our appreciation of what causes cancer. Epidemiology studies of various human populations indicated that inorganic metals such as arsenic and nickel could cause cancer. This was subsequently confirmed in laboratory studies with animals. Various hormones are implicated in organ-specific cancer, such as breast cancer. Nutrition and diet also appear to be related to cancer, specifically high caloric intake. The grain contaminant aflatoxin $B_1$ is known to cause liver cancer. Chemical mixtures or exposure to multiple agents can increase the incidence of cancer, for example smoking and asbestos exposure increase the likelihood of lung cancer. And, finally, we are now learning that our genetic makeup increases the likelihood that certain cancers will develop. For example, breast cancer has been linked to specific genes.

Our cells and bodies have evolved to fight off cancer. Specific DNA repair mechanisms work to correct damaged DNA. Our immune system works to isolate and kill rogue cancer cells. Cancer appears to be part of life, an aspect of the aging process, even bad luck. Clearly, however, we have learned that reducing our exposure to certain chemical and physical agents can decrease the likelihood of developing cancer or at least delay its onset.

---

**Causes of cancer**
Organic chemicals (alcohol, tars, dyes, solvents . . . )
Inorganic agents (metals – arsenic, nickel . . . )
Hormones
Nutrition (diet, fat, high calories)
Chemical mixtures
Genetics

## 16.2 Case studies

### 16.2.1 Soot

In 1775, Percivall Pott observed that there was an increased incidence of cancer of the scrotum in chimney sweeps and suggested that soot may be the cause. This was the first linking of occupational chemical exposure to cancer. Unfortunately this understanding was not translated into action and prevention. By the late 1890s, scrotal cancer was relatively rare on the European content but still high in England, which some suggested was due to poor hygiene. Failure to remove the soot from the skin resulted in chronic exposure to the chemicals in soot, which resulted in cancer. It is back to the most basic tenets of public health – wash your hands (or other body parts). Scientific investigation of the cancer-causing properties of soot took a step forward when Japanese research found that skin tumors developed when coal tar was repeatedly applied to the skin of rabbits. In the 1930s, polycyclic aromatic hydrocarbon was isolated from coal tar and demonstrated to be carcinogenic. Despite this evidence, millions of people continue to expose themselves to the soot from tobacco and suffer from the resulting lung cancer.

### 16.2.2 Benzene

Benzene, $C_6H_6$, is a clear, colorless liquid at room temperature and readily evaporates into the air. It is derived from petroleum and is widely used in the production of other products such as rubber, nylon, synthetic fibers, lubricants, glues, detergents, dyes, drugs, and pesticides, to name just a few. Worldwide, benzene use and production are measured in the billions of pounds, making it one of the top 20 chemicals in use. In the United States, benzene is present in gasoline at about 2%, but in other countries may be up to 5%. It is readily absorbed by inhalation. Acute exposure can result in central nervous system effects such as dizziness, drowsiness, and eventual unconscious. Liver enzymes convert benzene to more toxic metabolites, which is thought to be the mechanism for the carcinogenic effects of benzene. Chronic exposure to benzene affects the bone marrow by crippling blood cell production, causing anemia, which can ultimately result in leukemia. At one time benzene was widely used as a solvent, resulting in excessive worker exposure; it continues to be a significant workplace contaminant. Benzene is present in the indoor environment from out-gassing of glues, synthetic materials, and tobacco smoke. Smokers can have benzene body burdens 10 times that of nonsmokers. Because of its widespread use in industry, benzene is a common contaminant of hazardous waste and old industrial sites. The US EPA recommends that benzene not exceed 5 ppb (parts per billion or 0.005 mg/l) in drinking water. The US Occupational Health and Safety Administration set a standard of 1 ppm of benzene in the air over an 8-hour period with an action level set at 0.5 ppm in an effort to encourage reductions in the workplace environment. Other agencies have established even lower standards down to 0.1 ppm benzene in the air.

### 16.2.3 Asbestos

Asbestos, a recognized human carcinogen, has a long and curious history. Asbestos continues to cause serious human health effects and continues to be the subject of legal action against companies that used or produced it. Asbestos is the common name given to a group of six different naturally occurring fibrous minerals that can be separated into long fibers, spun, and woven. The material is strong, flexible, resistant to heat and most solvents and acids, making it a very desirable industrial product. Knowledge of asbestos goes back to the second century BC, but the first recorded use of the word asbestos was in the first century AD by Pliny the Elder. The fire-resistant properties of asbestos were recognized early and contributed to its derivation from the Greek *sbestos* or extinguishable, thus a-sbestos or inextinguishable. The Romans used asbestos to make cremation cloths and lamp wicks and, in the Middle Ages, knights used asbestos to insulate their suits of armor. The use of asbestos increased along with the Industrial Revolution and the need for a material to insulate steam boilers, such as those in locomotives.

The first asbestos mine opened in 1879 in Quebec, Canada. Canada continues to be the world's largest producer of asbestos, followed by Russia, China, Brazil, and several other countries. In the United States, California produces a small amount, but the majority of the asbestos used in the United States is imported from Canada. Serious lung disease associated with asbestos inhalation was first described in the early 1900s in England. This disease became known as asbestosis and was fully described in British medical journals in 1924 as young workers died from asbestos exposure. By the early 1930s, dose-related injury, length of time exposed, and the latency to response were being well characterized in both Europe and the United States. By the mid- to late 1930s the first associations with lung cancer were documented. In the 1960s the consequences of asbestos exposure for many workers in the Second World War started to become evident. Mesothelioma, a cancer of the lining of the lung, was found to be almost exclusively associated with asbestos exposure. In the United States regulation of asbestos exposure stated in the early 1970s with exposure limits rapidly decreasing as the serious and latent consequences of asbestos exposure became apparent. White asbestos or chrysotile was used in thousands of consumer products and is common in many older homes. The serious health effects of asbestos exposure have resulted in both regulatory and legal action and in many countries the total banning of the use of asbestos.

### 16.2.4 Radon

Radon is another example of a very curious and toxic compound that many of us regularly inhale, hopefully in small amounts. For those regularly exposed to radon, there is an increased risk for lung cancer and, for those that smoke, radon exposure results in a three-fold increase in the incidence of lung cancer. In the United States it is estimated that indoor radon exposure causes between 7000 and 30,000 lung cancer-related deaths each year, second only to tobacco smoking. Radon-222 is a colorless and odorless radioactive gas that results from the decay of radium-226, which is widely distributed in the earth's crust. Radon decays with a half-life of 3.8 days into solid particles of polonium. It is actually the breakdown of polonium that causes cancer. Polonium sticks to the tissues of the lung, and when it decays, an alpha particle is released which damages the DNA of the closest cell, ultimately causing lung cancer. Lung diseases, possibly related to radon, were first reported in the 1400s, and in 1879 lung cancer was seen in European miners. Radon was discovered several years later in 1900 by the German chemist Friedrich Ernst Dorn. Regulation of workplace exposure began in the 1950s and subsequent studies of underground mineworkers in Canada, Czechoslovakia, France, Australia, Sweden, and the United States have allowed researchers to develop very sophisticated models of the cancer-causing effects of radon. It is difficult to translate these results into the effects of radon on indoor home exposure. The United States EPA sets an action level of four picocuries per liter (pCi/l). There are some areas of the United States and Europe with high levels of radon that can enter a home, school, or public building, particularly the below-ground levels. In the United States, it is estimated that 1 in 15 (6%) of homes have elevated levels of radon. A number of public and private organizations provide information on reducing indoor radon exposure.

## 16.3 Biology of cancer and genetic toxicology

Cancer is the result of a cell's machinery going horribly out of control. In its simplest form, there is a permanent change in a cell's DNA that allows that cell to divide repeatedly, passing this change along to the next cell. To understand cancer it is necessary to explore the cellular changes that turn a normal cell into a malignant cell that repeatedly and uncontrollably divides. This transformation occurs when there is genetic damage or an alteration in the structure of a cell's DNA.

Genetic toxicology is the study of effects of chemical and physical agents on genetic material. Genetic toxicology includes the study of DNA damage in living cells that leads to cancer, but also changes in DNA that can be inherited from one generation to the next. The relevance of genetic toxicology is clearly evident from inheritable diseases such as phenylketonuria (an inability to metabolize phenylalanine), cystic fibrosis (lung disease), sickle cell anemia, or Tay–Sachs disease. Recent advances in molecular biology and genomic sciences are leading to a far greater understanding of the genetic causes of disease and even pointing the way to treatments.

Genetic toxicology, although not called that at the time, started in 1927 when American geneticist Hermann J. Muller (1890–1967) demonstrated that X-rays increased the rate of gene mutations and chromosome changes in fruit flies. At that time Muller and others were investigating how naturally occurring changes in genes related to structural changes in the fruit fly. The rapidly reproducing and short-lived fruit fly was an excellent subject, but waiting for the spontaneous changes to occur in their genes (at that time they did not yet know about DNA) was slow. Muller used X-rays to increase the rate of change in genes, thus furthering his research efforts but also demonstrating an important toxicological property of X-rays. As our knowledge of biology deepened, it was discovered how the energy of X-rays caused changes in the DNA.

DNA, short for deoxyribonucleic acid, is the coding machinery of life. The beauty of DNA is in its simplicity that results in the complexity of life. The double helix of DNA is made of the chemicals adenine (A), guanine (G), thymine (T), and cytosine (C). These chemical are bound in long stretches as AT and CG pairs, and wrapped in sugar molecules to hold them together. Long stretches of these AT and CG combinations form genes which when "read" produce the proteins that drive our cells.

Typical short strand of DNA

**G C A G C A T**
**C G T C G T A**

When sequences of G, C, A, and T are read (by RNA), they are translated into other chemicals that eventually become proteins. Ideally the DNA sequence would not change except in the recombination that occurs during reproduction. However, a cell's DNA is located in the very dynamic and demanding environment of the cell, where damage can occur. DNA damage occurs regularly as part of the cell process and from interaction with normal cellular chemicals as well as toxic chemicals. Fortunately, there is a very robust repair mechanism that rapidly and very accurately repairs the DNA damage. However, if for some reason the DNA is repaired incorrectly, a mutation occurs. The mutation is a subtle or even not so subtle change in the A, G, C, or T that make up the DNA.

Normal strand of DNA – Mutated Strand

**G C A G C A T      G C A A C A T**
**C G T C G T A      C G T T G T A**

Many of the mutations have no effect, some have minor effects, and an even smaller number have life-threatening effects. If a mutation occurs in the wrong place, a cell can start to divide uncontrollably, becoming a malignant cell and causing a cancer. If a mutation occurs in our germ line cells it can be passed on to our offspring. Muller used X-rays to induce many mutations, some of which would be in the germ line cells of fruit fly and thus passed on to the next generation, which he could study.

Chemicals can damage the DNA and induce mutations. Chemicals that induce mutations in the DNA are called mutagens, and when these changes lead to cancer the chemical is called a carcinogen. Not all mutagens are carcinogens and not all carcinogens are mutagens, but in general it is best to avoid mutagens. In 1946 it was shown that nitrogen mustards (derived from mustard gas first used by the military in 1917 during the First World War) could induce mutations in the fruit fly and reduce tumor growth in mice. As the relationship of gene mutations to cancer become evident, genetic toxicology developed ways to test chemical and physical agents for their mutagenic properties. In the 1970s these tests were greatly simplified when Bruce Ames and others developed a cellular-based test for genetic mutations. This test became know as the Ames assay. Sophisticated variations of these tests are now required to assess the mutagenicity of a chemical before approval for use by many government regulatory agencies. For example, you would not want an artificial sweetener to cause mutations even at a very low rate.

Often it is not the parent compound that causes the cancer but a metabolite of the original compound. Ideally, a foreign chemical is made less toxic by metabolism, but sometimes a chemical can be made more toxic. This more toxic chemical can then interact with cellular DNA or proteins and produce malignant cells. This process is called bioactivation. It is also possible that another chemical may encourage bioactivation or possibly interact to accelerate the development of a cancer. This knowledge influences the tests required of chemicals because some were not mutagens until metabolized by liver enzymes. Many variations of the Ames test were developed that include liver cells to simulate the metabolism of the liver and determine if bioactivation would result in mutations.

Efforts to understand the underlying biology of cancer are ongoing. The genomic sciences are helping to explain why some people are more susceptible to cancer than others. We also know that there are many causes of cancer and that we can reduce the likelihood of developing cancer.

## 16.4 What causes cancer?

The causes of cancer are varied: many known, most likely multiple, many unknown, and just a random event of no specific cause. We are continuously exposed to a wide range of chemical and physical agents, from both natural and human generated sources that may cause cancer. Because our knowledge is not perfect there is a great deal of conflicting information on the causes of cancer and what can be done to reduce the risk of developing cancer. We are just beginning to understand how our individual genetic makeup influences the possibility of developing cancer and other genetic-based disease. In the future we will have even more knowledge about how the environment interacts with our genetics to cause cancer. We will briefly examine some of the known causes of cancer (Table 16.2).

Lifestyle choices are the cause of many cancers. This is obvious from even a quick look at the correlation between tobacco consumption and lung cancer. The age-adjusted incidence of lung cancer for males peaked in the late 1980s and then started to decline with the decline in smoking. But for females, the increase in lung cancer appears to be peaking in the late 1990s and has yet to start declining.

**Table 16.2 Exposure to cancer causing agents**

| Cause | Example |
|---|---|
| Lifestyle | Tobacco consumption – drinking – diet |
| Environmental exposures | Air, drinking water |
| Organic chemicals | Benzo(a)pyrene (coal tar), benzene |
| Inorganic chemicals | Arsenic, cadmium, nickel |
| Fibers | Asbestos |
| Radiation | Sun (ultraviolet), radioactive material |
| Drugs | DES (diethylstilbestrol) |
| Viruses | Epstein–Barr virus, AIDS, papillomavirus |
| Genetic | Increased likelihood (breast cancer) |

These data are testifying to the delayed onset of cancer and the relationship with tobacco consumption. Tobacco consumption probably accounts for between 25 and 40% of all cancer deaths.

The other major lifestyle choices associated with cancer are diet and alcohol consumption. Alcohol increases the incidence of liver disease and cancer. Diet has a broad range of effects, some good and some not so good. Some cooked meats have a higher concentration of agents that appear to cause cancer. On the other hand, a diet rich in vegetables may reduce the incidence of cancer. High caloric intake and high fat consumption may encourage the onset of cancer from other agents. As with most things, a high dose results in a greater response. In most cases a high dose of calories, fat, alcohol, or tobacco increases the likelihood of cancer.

Numerous organic chemical agents are known, or are highly likely, to cause cancer. In the 1930s benzo(a)pyrene was isolated from coal tar and shown to cause skin cancer. Further investigation discovered an entire class of carcinogenic compounds called polycyclic aromatic hydrocarbons (PAHs) that caused cancer. Prior to the Second World War there was a rich period of chemical synthesis. It was soon discovered that the azo dyes could also cause cancer. Naturally occurring contaminants from a grain fungus (aflatoxin) was found to be a potent liver carcinogen. A high incidence of liver cancer occurred when grain was poorly stored and people had liver disease such as hepatitis. People from hot and humid areas of Africa were particularly at risk for liver cancer form this grain fungus.

Inorganic chemicals and fibers may also be carcinogenic. Arsenic is the most serious human carcinogen because of exposure from drinking water (see arsenic chapter). Cadmium, chromium, and nickel are all lung carcinogens. The most common lung carcinogen is asbestos. The unique properties of asbestos made it ideal for many industrial and even home insulation applications. It was used in shipyards and in car brake pads. This widespread use resulted in thousand of workers being exposed to asbestos and suffering from a range of lung diseases including cancer. Asbestos exposure produces a very unique form of lung cancer called mesothelioma. Mesothelioma is caused in part by the fibers inducing a chronic irritation of the lung resulting in an inflammatory response that ultimately results in some cells becoming cancerous.

Hormones regulate many important bodily functions and are also associated with cancer. One of the first hints of the relationship of hormones to cancers was the observation that nuns had a greater incidence of breast cancer. This was naturally related to the nuns not having children and now we know that breast cancer may be hormone related. Since then there have been numerous studies on the use of birth control with cancer, childbirth, and most recently hormone replacement association with cancer. In males there is ongoing study of the hormones and prostate cancer. While it is clear that hormones and cancer are related, the exact characterization of this relationship is still unclear.

We are becoming increasingly aware of the importance of diet and nutrition in reducing the risk of cancer. From a toxicological perspective, it is important to reduce exposure to agents that increase the risk of cancer. Cancer, like declining physical and mental ability, is related to old age and may even be a natural consequence of the aging process. However, exposure to cancer-causing agents increases the risk or likelihood of developing cancer.

## 16.5 Who is vulnerable?

We are all vulnerable to cancer. Exposure to sunlight, background radiation, natural and manufactured chemicals, even oxygen can damage our DNA and result in cancer. We know that exposure to certain chemical or physical agents can increase the risk of developing cancer. There are many examples of workplace exposures resulting in cancer. Radon gas in coal and uranium mines can cause lung cancer. Asbestos exposure has affected thousands of workers and resulted in compensation claims from the companies. Of course, not smoking would result in the greatest reduction in cancers and other health-related effects of tobacco.

Figures 16.1 and 16.2 illustrate the US male and female cancer rates from 1938 to 1998. The most striking changes, for both male and female, are for lung cancer, which also reflects the changes in cigarette smoking. The peaks in lung cancer correspond to the delay in onset of lung cancer after the start of smoking. The incidence of lung cancer in males is declining with the drop in tobacco consumption, while that of females is just peaking.

Advances in the genomic sciences will ultimately provide us with individual knowledge of our vulnerability to cancer. Some of these cancers are triggered by interaction of genes and environmental exposures. This knowledge will provide even more incentive to reduce or control exposure to specific agents.

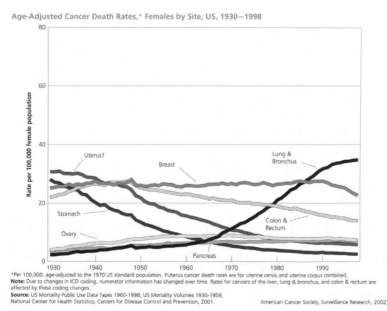

Age-Adjusted Cancer Death Rates,* Females by Site, US, 1930–1998

*Per 100,000, age-adjusted to the 1970 US standard population. †Uterus cancer death rates are for uterine cervix and uterine corpus combined.
**Note:** Due to changes in ICD coding, numerator information has changed over time. Rates for cancers of the liver, lung & bronchus, and colon & rectum are affected by these coding changes.
**Source:** US Mortality Public Use Data Tapes 1960-1998, US Mortality Volumes 1930-1959, National Center for Health Statistics, Centers for Disease Control and Prevention, 2001.

American Cancer Society, Surveillance Research, 2002

**Figure 16.1.** Female age-adjusted cancer death rates.
Source: Cancer Facts and Figure – 2002. Reprinted by the permission of the American Cancer Society, Inc.

Age-Adjusted Cancer Death Rates,* Males by Site, US, 1930–1998

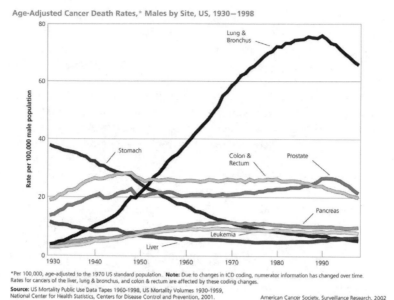

*Per 100,000, age-adjusted to the 1970 US standard population.  **Note:** Due to changes in ICD coding, numerator information has changed over time. Rates for cancers of the liver, lung & bronchus, and colon & rectum are affected by these coding changes.
**Source:** US Mortality Public Use Data Tapes 1960-1998, US Mortality Volumes 1930-1959, National Center for Health Statistics, Centers for Disease Control and Prevention, 2001.      American Cancer Society, Surveillance Research, 2002

**Figure 16.2.** Male age-adjusted cancer death rates.
Source: Cancer Facts and Figure – 2002. Reprinted by the permission of the American Cancer Society, Inc.

## 16.6 Regulatory standards

National and international agencies have established systems to classify agents according to the likelihood that the agent will cause cancer. This is often a difficult process because the information on an agent may be incomplete or inconclusive. Data from any human epidemiology studies are evaluated first and then information from animal studies. The International Agency for Research on Cancer (IARC) has developed one of the most comprehensive classification schemes. In this scheme an agent is rated from 1 to 4 based on human and animal data (Table 16.3).

Government regulatory agencies do not always agree on the classification of cancer-causing compounds and there are several different schemes used by different agencies. Elaborate animal study protocols are used to determine if an agent may cause cancer. As part of the approval process, government agencies require animal testing for carcinogenicity for new compounds entering the food supply. We want to be sure that the latest artificial sweetener will not cause cancer.

## 16.7 Recommendation and conclusions

The war on cancer is really a long and never ending battle. While scientists have made great strides in understanding the causes of cancer and developing treatments, there will always be a risk of developing cancer. As individuals we can be aware of the risks of exposure to suspected carcinogens and take appropriate actions to reduce our exposure. The likelihood of developing cancer is related to our individual

**Table 16.3 IARC classification scheme for human carcinogenicity**

| Group | Evidence | Examples |
|---|---|---|
| 1. Agent is human carcinogen | Sufficient human data | Aflatoxin, benzene, arsenic |
| 2A. Agent is probably a human carcinogen | Limited human data Sufficient animal data | PCBs, styrene oxide |
| 2B. Agent is possibly a human carcinogen | Limited or inadequate human data Sufficient animal data | Styrene, TCDD |
| 3. Agent is not classifiable as a human carcinogen | Not enough human or animal data | Diazepam |
| 4. Agent is probably not a human carcinogen | Inadequate human data Inadequate animal data | |

sensitivity and our dose–response curve. Less exposure means you will be less likely to develop cancer.

## 16.8 More information and references

### 16.8.1 Slide presentation

■ A Small Dose of Cancer and Genetic Toxicology presentation material. Online. Available HTTP: <http://www.crcpress.com/e_products/> and follow the links to downloads and then the catalog number TF1691.

### 16.8.2 European, Asian, and international agencies

■ IARC – International Agency for Research on Cancer (IARC) – World Health Organization (WHO). Online. Available HTTP: <http://www.iarc.fr/> (accessed: 5 April 2003).
  IARC's mission is to coordinate and conduct research on the causes of human cancer, the mechanisms of carcinogenesis, and to develop scientific strategies for cancer control.
■ World Health Organization (WHO) – Cancer. Online. Available HTTP: <http://www.who.int/health_topics/cancer/en/> (accessed: 5 April 2003).
  Site has information on international exposure to a wide range of compounds that cause cancer.
■ Japan – National Cancer Center (English). Online. Available HTTP: <http://www.ncc.go.jp/index.html> (accessed: 5 April 2003).
  Site has information on the treatment and causes of cancer in Japan (Japanese or English version available).
■ Australia – SunSmart. Online. Available HTTP: <http://www.sunsmart.com.au/> (accessed: 5 April 2003).
  An Australian site that focuses on skin cancer, primarily caused by the sun.

■ Australia – Cancer Council Victoria. Online. Available HTTP: <http://www.cancervic.org.au/index.htm> (accessed: 6 April 2003).
"The Cancer Council Victoria is an independent, volunteer-based charity whose mission is to lead, coordinate, implement and evaluate action to minimise the human cost of cancer for all Victorians."

■ Asbestos Institute. Online. Available HTTP: <http://www.asbestos-institute.ca/> (accessed: 5 April 2003).
The Asbestos Institute is dedicated to promoting the safe use of asbestos in Canada and throughout the world. (French and English).

### 16.8.3 North American agencies

#### 16.8.3.1 General information on cancer

■ US Food and Drug Administration (FDA). Online. Available HTTP: <http://www.fda.gov/cder/cancer/index.htm> (accessed: 5 April 2003).
Oncology Tools contains a variety of information related to cancer and approved cancer drug therapies.

■ US Environmental Protection Agency (EPA). Online. Available HTTP: <http://www.epa.gov/ncea/cancer.htm> (accessed: 5 April 2003).
EPA cancer risk assessment guidelines.

■ US Environmental Protection Agency (EPA) – National Center for Environmental Assessment (NECA). Online. Available HTTP: <http://cfpub.epa.gov/ncea/> (accessed: 5 April 2003).
Applying science to improve risk assessment and environmental decision making.

■ US National Cancer Institute (NCI). Online. Available HTTP: <http://www.cancer.gov/> (accessed: 5 April 2003).
The NCI, established under the National Cancer Act of 1937, is the Federal Government's principal agency for cancer research and training.

■ US Centers for Disease Control and Prevention (CDC). Online. Available HTTP: <http://www.cdc.gov/cancer/> (accessed: 5 April 2003).
The CDC monitors cancer incidence and promotes cancer prevention and control.

■ US National Cancer Institute – The Cancer Mortality Maps & Graph Web Site. Online. Available HTTP: <http://www3.cancer.gov/atlasplus/> (accessed: 5 April 2003).
This site provides interactive maps, graphs (which are accessible to the blind and visually-impaired), text, tables, and figures showing geographic patterns and time trends of cancer death rates for the time period 1950–1994 for more than 40 cancers.

■ US Cancer Information Service (CSI). Online. Available HTTP: <http://cis.nci.nih.gov/> (accessed: 5 April 2003).
A service of the US National Cancer Institute, CSI, is a "source for the latest, most accurate cancer information for patients, their families, the general public, and health professionals".

■ US Brookhaven National Laboratory – Safety & Health Services Chemical Management. Online. Available HTTP: <http://www.bnl.gov/esh/shsd/cms/Safety_Carcinogens.htm> (accessed: 5 April 2003).

Site contains a comprehensive table listing chemicals and compares their designation as carcinogens by national and international agencies.

### 16.8.3.2 Benzene information

- US Environmental Protection Agency (EPA). Online. Available HTTP: <http://www.epa.gov/ttn/atw/hlthef/benzene.html> (accessed: 5 April 2003).
  Hazard fact sheet on benzene.
- US Agency for Toxic Substance Disease Registry (ATSDR). Online. Available HTTP: <http://www.atsdr.cdc.gov/> (accessed: 5 April 2003).
  See fact sheets and case studies in environmental medicine (benzene).

### 16.8.3.3 Asbestos information

- US Environmental Protection Agency (EPA). Online. Available HTTP: <http://www.epa.gov/opptintr/asbestos/> (accessed: 5 April 2003).
  Extensive information on asbestos.
- US Cancer Information Service (CSI) – Facts of Asbestos. Online. Available HTTP: <http://cis.nci.nih.gov/fact/3_21.htm> (accessed: 5 April 2003).
  Extensive information on asbestos.

### 16.8.3.4 Radon information

- US Environmental Protection Agency (EPA). Online. Available HTTP: <http://www.epa.gov/iaq/radon/> (accessed: 5 April 2003).
  USEPA has extensive information on radon exposure in the US.
- US Geological Survey (USGS). Online. Available HTTP: <http://energy.cr.usgs.gov/radon/radonhome.html> (accessed: 5 April 2003).
  Maps and supply information on radon in the United States.

## 16.8.4 Non-government organizations

- The American Cancer Society (ACS). Online. Available HTTP: <http://www.cancer.org/> (accessed: 5 April 2003).
  The ACS is a nationwide community-based voluntary health organization dedicated to eliminating cancer as a major health problem by preventing cancer, saving lives, and diminishing suffering from cancer, through research, education, advocacy, and service.
- Asbestos Network. Online. Available HTTP: <http://www.asbestosnetwork.com/index.htm> (accessed: 5 April 2003).
  A legal firm supports this site on "Asbestos: Mesothelioma, Asbestosis, and Other Problems" – good historical information.
- Boston University School of Public Health, Department of Environmental Health. Online. Available HTTP: <http://www.bumc.bu.edu/SPH/Gallery/> (accessed: 5 April 2003).
  This site has a very interesting article on the human side of asbestos exposure.

- The White Lung Association. Online. Available HTTP: <http://www.whitelung.org/> (accessed: 5 April 2003).
  Non-profit web site on asbestos exposure.
- National Radon Safety Board (NRSB). Online. Available HTTP: <http://www.nrsb.org/> (accessed: 5 April 2003).
  "The NRSB seeks to encourage the highest standards of practice and integrity in radon services through the development of independent standards and procedures for certifying, approving and accrediting radon testers, mitigators, measurement devices, chambers and laboratories."
- American Lung Association (ALA). Online. Available HTTP: <http://www.lungusa.org/air/envradon.html> (accessed: 5 April 2003).
  Site has information on radon in the home environment as well as tobacco and asthma.
- Environmental Mutagen Society (EMS). Online. Available HTTP: <http://www.ems-us.org/> (accessed: 5 April 2003).
  EMS fosters research on the basic mechanisms of mutagenesis as well as on the application of this knowledge in the field of genetic toxicology.

# Chapter 17

# Pregnancy and developmental toxicology

## Contents

- Introduction and history
- Reproduction
- Pregnancy
- Development
- Examples
- Regulatory issues
- More information and references

## 17.1 Introduction and history

Nature creates monsters for the purpose of astonishing us and amusing herself.
Pliny (AD 61–105)

Life evolves through sexual reproduction and the development of the resulting organism. It is truly astonishing that male and female germ cells (a sperm and an egg) can merge and develop into an independent organism. In order to facilitate the discussion of this enormous and complex subject, it will be divided into three areas: reproduction – issues associated with the egg and sperm; pregnancy – the critical environment of early development; and development of the infant. The focus will be primarily on humans, but the development of all organisms can be adversely affected by chemical or physical agents. The chapter provides only the briefest examination of the disorders and adverse effects of various agents on reproduction and development. Harmful agents affect the developing organism in dramatic and subtle ways and that can harm a person for a lifetime at enormous cost to the individual and society.

Only in the last 100 years have we begun to understand the mysteries of reproduction and development. Prior to advances in the biological sciences, ancient civilization invoked a fertility goddess to oversee reproduction. Many thought malformed or abnormal infants were a message or warning of future events. A small statue of conjoined twins dating from 6500 BC was discovered in Turkey. A clay tablet (2000 BC) found along the Tigris River described 62 malformations and related the abnormalities to future events. In the fifteenth and sixteenth centuries, malformed infants were thought to be a product of the devil and both mother and child were killed. Some thought that the development of the child was influenced by what the mother was viewing. Thus, Aristotle recommended that a mother view beautiful statuary to increase her child's beauty. One definition of the word monster is an abnormal animal or plant. Monster is derived from the Latin *monstrum omen*, and from *monere* to warn, reflecting the notion that abnormal infants told of the future. Greek for monster is *teras*, which is the route of teratology, the study of malformations or monsters.

The more scientific investigation of abnormal development began in the 1830s when Etienne Geoffroy Saint-Hilaire studied the effects of different conditions on the development of chicken eggs. However, it was not until the late 1800s and early 1900s that it was more widely recognized that genetics played an important role in development. In the 1930s and 1940s, experiments by Josef Warkany and others clearly demonstrated that a wide range of agents such as vitamin A deficiency, nitrogen mustard, alkylating agents, hypoxia, and X-rays could cause malformation in rodents. In 1941, the rubella virus infection was linked to malformed infants. However, many thought that the placental environment protected the infant during pregnancy. This understanding changed dramatically with the discovery that methyl mercury was a developmental toxicant and in the 1960s when thalidomide caused severe abnormalities (see below).

While the knowledge that toxic agents can dramatically affect the developing fetus has only developed relatively recently, there is a long and curious history of toxicology and reproduction. Since ancient times, people have sought ways to stop the onset of reproduction by killing the sperm before they meet the egg. A variety of natural products were used with varying degrees of success. Now, more modern chemicals specifically designed to be toxic to sperm, such as nonoxynol-9, are used as a spermicides. There is ongoing effort to develop compounds that are not toxic to people but are toxic to the viruses and bacteria that cause sexually transmitted diseases.

Continuing advances in the biological sciences as well as technology provided greater insight into the reproductive process. This research developed into a detailed understanding of the hormones that control the female reproductive process. In the 1950s and 1960s, "the pill" was developed that manipulated the natural estrogen and progesterone hormones and thus the onset of the reproductive process. Early versions of "the pill" had a number of undesirable side effects, which reduced when the drug levels were lowered. In essence, "the pill" is an endocrine disruptor and a desirable one. It was subsequently discovered that many different chemicals could affect the endocrine system. Some of these chemicals, such as DDT and dioxin, were widely distributed in the environment and began to reduce the fertility of wildlife.

We will now examine in more detail some of the physiological and toxicological aspects of reproduction, pregnancy, and development.

## 17.2 Reproduction

For all species, reproduction is essential, and most cases start with the merging of the egg and sperm cells. In humans, it is estimated that 50% of all pregnancies end in miscarriage or spontaneous abortion, often before the woman realizes that she is pregnant. The most common reason for a pregnancy to fail is chromosomal abnormality. Human cells have 46 chromosomes, which are the genes that control cell function and make us unique. The egg and the sperm cells contain only 23 chromosomes and must correctly combine during reproduction to create a cell with 46 chromosomes and start the development process. Failures in this process and the early stages of cell division are thought to be the primary reason for early loss of pregnancy.

Successful reproduction (and sex) involves many complex chemical processes that can be disrupted at various points to reduce fertility and conception. Part of this process is under control of the endocrine system, and chemicals that affect the endocrine system are termed endocrine disruptors. In the 1950s, understanding of the endocrine system led to the development of birth control pills as a way to reduce fertility in humans. This is a desirable and planned use of endocrine disruptors. Subsequently, it was discovered that a number of chemicals released into the environment could disrupt the endocrine system and reduce fertility of wildlife. Some are concerned that exposure to these chemicals, such as DDT and dioxin (TCDD), may also affect human fertility (Table 17.1). Approximately 15% of couples of reproductive age are infertile. Endocrine disruptors may also affect fetal development, causing demasculization and feminization of the offspring, which in turn cause reduced fertility in the next generation.

Chemicals can also directly affect male reproductive organs or sperm. Decreased sperm count, decreased sperm motility, or abnormalities can result in male sterility or reduced fertility. For example, occupational exposure to lead can result in infertility due to sperm abnormalities. Male sterility can also result from exposure to the fungicide dibromochloropropane (DBCP). Drugs or chemicals, such as

### Table 17.1 Examples of chemicals that affect reproduction

| Class of chemical | Examples |
| --- | --- |
| Endocrine disruptors | DDT, dioxin |
| Heavy metals | Lead (decreased or abnormal sperm) |
| Organic Solvents | Toluene, benzene, n-hexane |
| Drugs | Alcohol, narcotics, hypotensive drugs, chemotherapeutic agents, steroids, diethylstilbestrol |
| Pesticides | Dibromochloropropane (DBCP), methoxychlor, linuron (herbicide) |
| Disease | Diabetes |

| Table 17.2 Physiological changes during pregnancy | |
| --- | --- |
| Cardiovascular | Increased cardiac output, heart rate, blood pressure, blood volume expands |
| Respiration | Oxygen consumption increases 15 to 20% |
| Urinary output | Increases |
| Gut absorption changes | Greater absorption of iron and calcium (or toxic compounds such as lead) |
| Liver metabolism | Decreases for some drugs or chemicals, i.e. caffeine (longer half-life) |

alcohol and narcotics, that affect the central nervous system can also reduce sexual activity and thus fertility.

Female reproductive organs are also vulnerable to the effects of chemicals, including changes in ovulation or menstrual cycle, decreased implantation of the fertilized egg, or inability to maintain pregnancy.

## 17.3 Pregnancy

The female body undergoes a number of significant changes during pregnancy, some of which can increase vulnerability to toxic compounds (Table 17.2). A healthy woman readily adapts to the chances of pregnancy, but it is important to be aware of the consequences of some of these changes. As the pregnancy progresses, the heart rate increases, the volume of blood circulating increases, and blood pressure increases. The expanded blood volume results in increased urinary output. Antibiotic prescriptions may need to be altered to accommodate the changes in blood volume and urinary excretion. Respiration is affected as oxygen consumption increases by 15 to 20%. Increased nutrients such as iron and calcium are required during pregnancy, and the gastrointestinal tract changes to increase absorption of selected nutrients. An unintended consequence of this change is an increased absorption of lead during pregnancy. Normally, the adult absorbs 10% of lead following oral exposure, but because lead substitutes for calcium, the lead absorption is increased to become more similar to that of a child. Liver function decreases, resulting in the decreased metabolism of certain drugs (an increase in half-life). For example, the metabolism of caffeine decreases during the second and third trimesters of pregnancy, resulting in higher blood caffeine levels for longer periods of time. The half-life of caffeine in a woman approximately doubles during pregnancy. Caffeine and its metabolites readily cross the placenta, exposing the infant to these chemicals.

## 17.4 Development

One of the great lessons learned in the past 50 years is that the developing organism is more vulnerable to the effects of many chemicals than the adult. This sensitivity begins at the time of fertilization and continues throughout childhood.

This knowledge has been reinforced numerous times through tragic experience with thalidomide, alcohol, methyl mercury, lead, and many other agents. Our knowledge has progressed from concern only over chemicals that cause physical fetal malformation to recognition that chemicals can cause much more subtle but still harmful effects.

A primary reason for the sensitivity of the developing fetus is the rapidly multiplying number of cells. Not only are the cells rapidly dividing, they are changing into organ-specific cells. The nervous system alone ultimately has over 100 billion nerve cells responsible for transmitting information, as well as over 1 trillion glial or connecting cells. Many of these cells will undergo migration to different regions of the brain, formation of synaptic connections with other cells, and some will even die off in a programmed manner. Throughout gestation, different organs or cells within an organ are going through various growth and development phases. Chemicals can interfere with this process in very unexpected and unpredictable ways.

The infant remains vulnerable to exposure to chemicals following birth. The infant's liver only gradually begins to function after about six months of age. This delay has important implications if the infant is exposed to drugs dependent on liver metabolism. For example, an infant cannot metabolize caffeine. The infant can only excrete the caffeine in the urine, resulting in the half-life of caffeine being measured in days rather than hours, as it would be for an adult. Infants are also growing rapidly and require nutrients such as calcium and iron, which are readily absorbed from the gastrointestinal tract. Lead, a well-established neurotoxicant, is absorbed along with the calcium, making the infant more vulnerable to any lead exposure. Infants will absorb 50% of lead from oral exposure while adults only absorb 10%. Infants are also much smaller than adults, so that even a small bout of exposure represents a large dose. The hand to mouth behavior of an infant increases exposure to contaminants that may be in household dust or on toys. In addition, infants have a higher respiratory rate and consume more food relative to their body weight. All these and other factors combine to increase an infant's vulnerability to harmful chemicals. Table 17.3 lists just a few of the compounds known to affect fetal and infant development.

### Table 17.3 Agents and chemicals that affect the developing infant

| | |
|---|---|
| Metals | Lead, methyl mercury, arsenic (in animals) |
| Chemicals | Chlorobiphenyls, solvents (toluene), endocrine disruptors (DDT, TCDD) |
| Radiation | X-rays (therapeutic), atomic fallout |
| Infections | Rubella virus, herpes simplex virus, toxoplasmosis, syphilis |
| Medical drugs | Antibiotics (tetracyclines), anticancer drugs, anticonvulsants (valproic acid), lithium, retinoids (vitamin A), thalidomide, diethylstilbestrol (DES), anticoagulants (warfarin) |
| Recreational drugs | Alcohol (ethanol), tobacco, cocaine, solvent abuse |
| Plants | Many herbs, skunk cabbage (*Veratrum californicum*) in sheep and cattle, parasites in frogs |

## 17.5 Examples

### 17.5.1 Thalidomide

Thalidomide was introduced in 1956 as a sedative (sleeping pill) and to reduce nausea and vomiting during pregnancy. It was withdrawn in 1961 after it was found to be a human teratogen. In 1960 researchers in Australia and Germany observed an unusual increase in rare human malformations of missing limbs (amelia) or shortened long bones (phocomelia), particularly of the arms. It was soon realized that these unusual malformations were associated with the consumption of thalidomide during early pregnancy. Over 5000 infants were affected by thalidomide, primarily in Europe, Canada, and Australia. There were very few cases in the United States because a reviewer at the US Food and Drug Administration, Frances Kelsey, demanded additional safety data prior to approval of thalidomide. The routine animal safety studies of that period had failed to predict the adverse effects of thalidomide. This event resulted in significant changes to the animal testing requirements to evaluate the possible teratogenic and developmental effects of drugs. Recently, thalidomide was approved to treat multiple myeloma and leprosy, but with extraordinary precautions being taken because of its developmental effects.

### 17.5.2 Ethanol (alcohol)

> You will conceive and bear a son . . . now then be careful to take no wine or strong drink and to eat nothing unclean.
>
> Bible, Judges 13:3–4.

The Bible (Judges 13:3–4) cautioned against the consumption of alcohol during pregnancy, but it was not until the 1970s that tragic fetal effects of alcohol were described in detail. Fetal alcohol syndrome (FAS), characterized by facial malformations, growth retardation, small head, and greatly reduced intelligence, results from maternal consumption of alcohol. FAS affects 4000 to 12,000 newborn infants per year in the United States and from 1 to 3 births per 1000 worldwide per year. A milder form of the developmental effects of alcohol is fetal alcohol effect (FAE). FAE infants are slow to develop and have learning disabilities. FAE affects up to 36,000 infants in the United States, while the number of infants affected worldwide is not known. Alcohol consumption during pregnancy is the most common preventable cause of adverse nervous system development. Alcohol should not be consumed during pregnancy in any amount.

### 17.5.3 Methyl mercury

Bacteria convert mercury (quick silver) to methyl mercury ($CH_3$-Hg) in an effort to detoxify the mercury. Other organisms, including fish, consume the bacteria along with the methyl mercury. Larger fish consume the smaller fish and accumulate methyl mercury in muscle. Humans and other animals consume the fish and can be poisoned by the mercury. The developing fetus is particularly sensitive to the adverse developmental effects of methyl mercury. The tragic effects of fetal methyl mercury exposure were first observed in the 1950s in Minamata, Japan. High exposure and severe developmental effects were observed in other unfortunate incidents including the consumption of seed grain coated with organic mercury in Iraq. Further study revealed that even low levels of methyl mercury exposure may harm the developing fetus. Across the globe there are advisories on fish consumption related to methyl mercury for children and women of childbearing age. This is an unfortunate development because fish are an excellent source of protein and essential fats.

### 17.5.4 Lead

The use of lead in paint and as a gasoline additive was one of the greatest public health disasters of the twentieth century. The Greek physician Dioscorides reported in the second century BC that "Lead makes the mind give way". In 1922 the League of Nations banned white-lead interior paint, a move which the United States declined to follow, and a year later leaded gasoline went on sale in the United States. Our experience with lead emphasizes the sensitivity and vulnerability of the developing nervous system. Not only is the developing nervous system more sensitive to lead, but children absorb more lead than adults following oral exposure and their small size means they receive a larger dose of lead. It is now well accepted that even low levels of lead exposure harm the developing nervous system, reducing the IQ for a lifetime. Regulatory authorities around the world are working to reduce lead exposure by removing lead from gasoline and removing lead-based paint.

### 17.5.5 Endocrine-disrupting chemicals

Depending upon the circumstance and desired effects, endocrine-disrupting chemicals can be either good or bad. The endocrine system is a finely balanced system responsible for fertility and many of the feminine and masculine traits we are all familiar with. Endocrine disruptors are used by millions of women in the form of "the pill" to control fertility. Chemicals in birth control pills subtly manipulate the endocrine system to reduce fertility. Unfortunately, we now know that many chemicals are capable of influencing the endocrine systems. When these chemicals, such as DDT and TCDD, are released into the environment, they reduce the fertility of wildlife. Exposure to endocrine disruptors is linked to decreased fertility in shellfish, fish, birds, and mammals. Endocrine disruptors such as nonylphenol have been shown to feminize male fish, interfering with reproduction. Some studies have also linked exposure to endocrine disruptors to decreases in human male sperm count. Ironically, urinary metabolites of the birth control pill as well as the female hormone estrogen pass through waste treatment plants and are released into the aquatic environment, where even small concentrations cause feminization of male fish.

### 17.5.6 Herbal medicines during pregnancy

Herbal or "natural" remedies are a multibillion dollar business that is largely unregulated by government agencies. Herbal products are readily available and are claimed to improve health, but they also contain many physiologically active chemicals. The ingredients have not undergone the rigorous testing required of medical drugs to determine if there are any undesirable effects on the developing fetus or infant. There is a long history of herbal remedies being used as contraceptives, to induce abortions, or to delay or increase uterine contractions. Any of these possible effects indicate that the herbal product should not be consumed during pregnancy. Manufacturers are not required to demonstrate safety of herbal or "natural" products. Given the sensitivity of the developing fetus, consumption of herbal products during pregnancy should be approached very cautiously.

## 17.6 Regulatory issues

Government regulatory authorities in Europe, North America, and Asia require extensive testing of food additives and new drugs for reproductive and developmental effects. A significant expansion of drug testing occurred following the tragic experience with thalidomide. Testing requirements have gradually evolved, becoming more sophisticated with our increased understanding of potential effects on the nervous system. Reproductive and developmental testing is also required of some pesticides and other chemicals that may be released into the environment or have significant human exposure.

A variety of cell-based and animal-based studies can be performed to ensure that a new chemical does not cause reproductive or developmental effects. A battery of tests is done to ensure that there are no harmful effects on fertility. Teratogenicity studies are performed to ensure that the chemical does not cause physical malformations in the offspring from exposure during pregnancy. Multiple generations of animals may be continuously exposed to ensure that a compound is safe.

There are an estimated 50,000 to 60,000 industrial chemicals in common use. We know very little about the reproductive and developmental effects of the majority of these chemicals. In addition, there are no safety testing requirements for "natural" products. In 1986, the voters of the State of California passed a law requiring the Governor of the state "to publish, at least annually, a list of chemicals known to the state to cause cancer or reproductive toxicity". This effort is an excellent source of information on chemicals that can cause birth defects or reproductive harm.

## 17.7 More information and references

### 17.7.1 Slide presentation

■   A Small Dose of Pregnancy and Developmental Toxicology presentation material. Online. Available HTTP: <http://www.crcpress.com/e_products/> and follow the links to downloads and then the catalog number TF1691.
    Web site contains presentation material related to this book for each chapter.

### 17.7.2 European, Asian, and international agencies

■   European Teratology Society (ETS). Online. Available HTTP: <http://www.etsoc.com/> (accessed: 1 April 2003).

The society is dedicated to the prevention of adverse effects on reproduction and development.

■ The Thalidomide Victims Association of Canada. Online. Available HTTP: <http://www.thalidomide.ca> (accessed: 30 March 2003).
Information on thalidomide in English or French.

### 17.7.3 North American agencies

■ US Food and Drug Administration – Center for Drug Evaluation and Research (CDER) – Thalidomide. Online. Available HTTP: <http://www.fda.gov/cder/news/thalinfo/default.htm> (accessed: 30 March 2003).
FDA information on their approval of thalidomide for treatment of leprosy.

■ Center for the Evaluation of Risks to Human Reproduction (CERHR) – The National Toxicology Program. Online. Available HTTP: <http://cerhr.niehs.nih.gov/> (accessed: 5 April 2003).
CERHR web site has "information about potentially hazardous effects of chemicals on human reproduction and development."

■ US National Library of Medicine – Current Bibliographies in Medicine 97–4 – Thalidomide: Potential Benefits and Risks. Online. Available HTTP: <http://www.nlm.nih.gov/pubs/cbm/thalidomide.html> (accessed: 30 March 2003).
The NLM site contains an extensive bibliography on thalidomide.

■ US Food and Drug Administration – Center for Food Safety and Applied Nutrition – Information for Pregnant Women Online. Available HTTP: <http://vm.cfsan.fda.gov/~dms/wh-preg.html> (accessed: 30 March 2003).
This FDA web site contains extensive information for pregnant women.

■ US National Women's Health Information Center – Center for Food Safety and Applied Nutrition – Information for Pregnant Women. Online. Available HTTP: <http://www.4woman.gov/Pregnancy/index.htm> (accessed: 30 March 2003).
Site contains general information on pregnancy and fetal development.

■ US Department of Health and Human Services – healthfinder – Information for Pregnant Women. Online. Available HTTP: <http://www.healthfinder.gov/scripts/SearchContext.asp?topic=688&refine=1> (accessed: 30 March 2003).
Site contains general information and links on pregnancy and fetal development for men and women.

■ US Centers for Disease Control and Prevention (CDC) – Health Topic: Pregnancy. Online. Available HTTP: <http://www.cdc.gov/health/pregnancy.htm> (accessed: 30 March 2003).
Site contains information and links on pregnancy and fetal development.

■ California – Office of Environmental Health Hazard Assessment – Proposition 65. Online. Available HTTP: <http://www.oehha.ca.gov/prop65.html> (accessed: 10 April 2003).
Passed in 1986 by the voters of California, Proposition 65 "requires the Governor to publish, at least annually, a list of chemicals known to the state to cause cancer or reproductive toxicity".

### 17.7.4 Non-government organizations

- Teratology Society. Online. Available HTTP: <http://teratology.org/> (accessed: March 30, 2003).
  "The Teratology Society is a multidisciplinary scientific society founded in 1960, the members of which study the causes and biological processes leading to abnormal development and birth defects at the fundamental and clinical level, and appropriate measures for prevention."
- Society for Developmental Biology. Online. Available HTTP: <http://sdb.bio.purdue.edu/> (accessed: 1 April 2003).
  "The purpose of the Society is to further the study of development in all organisms."
- March of Dimes. Online. Available HTTP: <http://www.modimes.org> (accessed: 1 April 2003).
  "March of Dimes works to "give all babies a fighting chance against the threats to their health: prematurity, birth defects, low birth weight"."

### 17.7.5 References

- Riddle, J. M. (1999). *Eve's Herbs: A History of Contraception and Abortion in the West.* Harvard University Press, Cambridge, Mass., 352 pp.

# Part 3

## Applied toxicology

# Chapter 18

## Toxics in the home

## Contents

- Dossier
- Introduction
- Exposure
- Risk
- Risk reduction
- Safer alternatives
- Recommendations
- More information and references

### 18.1 Dossier

**Name:** toxics in the home

**Use:** naturally occurring (mold, radon) and purchased household products (medicines, pesticides, cleaning agents, paint, mercury thermometers)

**Source:** natural and manufactured

**Recommended daily intake:** usually not recommended

**Absorption:** skin, oral, inhalation

**Sensitive individuals:** children (account for majority of poisoning incidents around the home)

**Toxicity/symptoms:** varies greatly (acute and long term effects)

**Regulatory facts:** EPA, FDA, Consumer Product Safety Commission

**General facts:** many household products are necessary, but often less toxic alternatives are available

**Environmental:** serious environmental concern (i.e. mercury, detergents)

**Recommendations:** use less toxic alternatives, dispose of hazardous wastes properly

## 18.2 Introduction

The home is a complex environment that contains many hazards and toxic materials, some naturally occurring and many others that we bring into the home. A common naturally occurring hazard is radon, a radioactive material that is released from the soil and bedrock. In a humid environment, mold and mildew can grow, releasing spores and toxins into the indoor air. Dust mites, invisible to the human eye, roam our home and in the right circumstances cause health problems. Some of the greatest hazards are from what we bring into the home.

The toxicology of household products is fascinating because it deals with products that we are all familiar with and because so many different kinds of products are involved. A typical home may contain cleaning products, cosmetics and personal care products, paints, medications, pesticides, fuels, and various solvents. Thermometers and thermostats may contain mercury, a well-known toxicant. Older homes were often painted with a lead-based paint, which if consumed causes serious developmental effects. Building materials may contain toxic solvents that are released into the home. The toxicity and ingredients of household products vary widely, but highly toxic products are found in most homes (Table 18.1).

Both the general environment and individuals in the home can suffer the consequences of the products used in and around the home. Many household products contain chemicals that when used contaminate our air and water. Consumers in the United States use about 8.3 billion pounds of dry laundry detergent and about a billion gallons of liquid detergent per year. Some of these laundry and dishwashing detergents contain phosphate. High phosphate levels in water encourage the growth of algae, which can suffocate other marine life. Mercury from broken thermometers can harm the individual but also moves into the atmosphere, into the water supply, and ultimately into the fish we eat. Paints, varnishes, motor oil, pesticides, antifreeze, and fluorescent lights are clearly hazardous wastes that when improperly disposed of harm the environment. Consumers in the United States generate 1.6 million tons of household hazardous waste each year. How many pounds of hazardous waste do you have in your home?

Many countries and regions have poison centers that provide information for people exposed to toxic substances. It is estimated that there are over 17,000 chemicals found in the home, many with only limited toxicity information. The centers maintain large databases on products and substances as well as the appropriate response

---

### Table 18.1 Toxics in the home

Radon
Lead in paint
Indoor air
Second-hand smoke
Mold and mildew
Household waste
Household products:
    Cleaning products, cosmetics and personal care products, paints, medications,
    pesticides, fuels, and various solvents, mercury-based thermometers

following exposure. Every day there are many household exposure incidents, some resulting in immediate and serious consequences (see box). By far, the most vulnerable population is children. In the United States more than 50% of poisoning incidents involve children less than six years of age. The poison centers primarily focus on acute or immediate response to an incident.

---

Poisoning events in United States – 2000
- 2.2 million reported exposures
- 53% involved children under age 6
- 90% occurred in the home
- 475,079 treated in a health-care facility
- 920 deaths reported in 2000

Source: National Poison Centers, 2000 data (Litovitz *et al.*, 2001)

---

Exposure to hazardous substances in the home can also have long-term health implications. Children and the elderly spend a great amount of time in the home, increasing their exposure to any toxic substances. Over 15 million people in the United States suffer from asthma, including 5 million children. The number of children with asthma continues to increase despite ongoing research into the possible causes. The causes may include household dust, droppings from dust mites, and mold. Asthma-related illness resulted in over 100,000 children visiting a hospital and losing over 10 million school days. A very different kind of long-term disability results from childhood lead exposure. The US Centers of Disease Control estimated that over one million US children have elevated blood lead levels due to household exposures.

## 18.3 Exposure

### 18.3.1 Routes of exposure

Residents can be exposed to household products by accidental ingestion, skin contact, splashing into the eyes, and by inhalation of vapors or airborne particles. Exposures can be short-term, resulting from a single product use or spill, to long-term, from frequent product use or off-gassing of volatile components.

---

Ingestion
 Direct ingestion of product
 Hand to mouth contact
Inhalation
 Acute inhalation of product during use
 Chronic inhalation of indoor air
Skin/eye contact
 Splashing/spilling during use
 Violent chemical reactions
 Contact with treated surfaces

---

### 18.3.2 Acute exposures

In the year 2000, poison centers in the United States responded to nearly two and half million incidents, mostly home exposures to chemical products, animal bites, and poisonous plants. Over 50% involved children under the age of six. In all, 24,024 incidents resulted in medical outcomes deemed "major", and there were 1711 deaths. Almost half (46%) stemmed from exposure to pharmaceutical products. Of the remaining exposures, the largest groups resulted from cosmetics and personal care products and household cleaners. Although the large number of incidents says more about the ubiquity of potentially hazardous products in the home than about their toxicity, the numbers also point out the extent of the potential dangers if products are toxic or if medical aid is not rapidly received. Many more deaths and serious injuries would occur if not for the rapid intervention of poison centers.

The following groups of household products can have serious and rapid acute health impacts.

#### 18.3.2.1 Corrosives

Strong acids, bases, or oxidizers can cause permanent eye damage, skin burns, and, if swallowed, gastrointestinal damage. Examples of corrosive products include alkaline drain cleaners and oven cleaners, acid-based toilet bowl cleaners and rust removers, concentrated disinfectants, and some concentrated pesticides, especially fungicides.

#### 18.3.2.2 Solvents

Products with a high percentage of solvents, such as oil-based paints, paint removers, fuels, lighter fluids, furniture polishes, and some pesticides can cause potentially fatal pneumonia if aspirated into the lungs as a result of accidental ingestion. If used in an unventilated space, they can also cause symptoms of acute intoxication, including dizziness, nausea, and in some cases nerve damage or other effects.

#### 18.3.2.3 Medications

Useful as prescribed, many medications are toxic and can be very dangerous if taken by someone other than the intended patient, especially a child, or if taken in too high a dose.

#### 18.3.2.4 Pesticides

Although many household pesticides are rather dilute, some are concentrated enough to be acutely toxic. They include concentrates of insecticides, fungicides, and some herbicides.

### 18.3.3 Chronic exposures/chronic effects

Chronic, or long-term exposures can occur through repeated use of a product or through contact with long-lasting residues in the air, soil, household surfaces, or dust. The EPA's TEAM (Total Exposure Assessment Methodology) studies found that levels of a dozen volatile organic compounds were two to five times higher indoors than outdoors, regardless of the geographic location of the home. When volatile products are used indoors, levels of chemicals in the air can exceed background by 1000 times or more and persist for a long time. Contaminated soil can be a major source of exposure, especially for children who play in it or put their hands in their mouths. In addition to isolated, elevated levels of contaminants from industrial sources, studies show consistently elevated levels of lead near the foundation of homes once painted with lead-based paint. Wooden decks built from treated lumber containing arsenic typically contaminate the soil beneath to levels far above background. Lead and other contaminants are carried into the home on shoes, where they are stored in house dust. Carpets can contain large reservoirs of dust that elude all but the most diligent vacuuming. House dust also can contain elevated levels of pesticides, combustion soot, nicotine, and allergens.

Products containing volatile ingredients, such as solvents, cause a general decline in indoor air quality when used inside the home. Volatile solvents often found in household products include those shown in Table 18.2. The last column shows permissible air concentrations of these solvents in occupational settings. The higher the number is, the less toxic the material.

Certain household products contain ingredients that can cause long-term or delayed chronic health effects such as cancer, reproductive effects, nervous system effects,

**Table 18.2 Volatile toxic chemicals**

| Ingredient | Product | Occupational exposure limits (ppm) |
| --- | --- | --- |
| Ethanol | Alcoholic beverages | 1000 |
| Acetone | Nail polish remover | 750 |
| Ethyl acetate | Nail polish remover, marker pens | 400 |
| Isopropanol | Rubbing alcohol, personal care products | 400 |
| Gasoline | Motor fuel | 300 |
| Methanol | Paint remover | 200 |
| Turpentine | Paint thinner | 100 |
| Xylene | Spray paint, market pens, adhesives | 100 |
| Hexane | Adhesives | 50 |
| Methylene chloride | Paint remover | 50 |
| Toluene | Paint remover, spray paints | 50 |
| Carbon monoxide | Vehicle exhaust, burning charcoal | 10 |
| Naphthalene | Mothballs | 10 |
| Paradichlorobenzene | Mothballs | 10 |
| Formaldehyde | Particle board, plywood | 0.30 |
| Chlorpyrifos | Insecticide* | 0.014 |

* Chlorpyrifos was discontinued in the US for household use after the end of 2001.

**Table 18.3 Chronic health effects**

| Ingredient | Found in | Cancer | Reproductive | Developmental | Nervous |
|---|---|---|---|---|---|
| Chlorothalonil | Fungicide | X | | | |
| Triforine | Fungicide | | | X | |
| Carbaryl | Insecticide | X | | | X |
| Arsenic | Treated wood | X | | | X |
| Lindane | Lice treatment | X | | | X |
| Paradichlorobenzene (PDCB) or naphthalene | Mothballs | X | | | |
| Hexane | Adhesive | | | | X |
| Lead acetate | Hair dye | X | X | X | X |
| Benzene | Gasoline | X | | X | |
| Aspirin | Pain relievers | | X | X | |
| Ethyl alcohol | Beverages | | | X | X |
| Methylene chloride | Paint remover | X | | | X |

and developmental effects. Table 18.3 lists some examples of types of products, ingredients, and the health effects that overexposure may lead to.

## 18.4 Risk

One of the greatest difficulties in estimating the toxicity of household products is the fact that most of the ingredients are not disclosed on product labels or other documents. Household pesticides, for example, often contain well over 90% so-called "inert" ingredients, more recently referred to as "other" ingredients. The terminology relates to their function in the product rather than their toxicological characteristics, and these ingredients, with few exceptions, are not listed on product labels. Although product labeling regulations in the United States do allow one to deduce certain acute toxicity characteristics from careful reading of required label warnings, the conclusions one can draw are limited. Frequently, the Material Safety Data Sheet (MSDS), a document required by the US. Occupational Safety and Health Administration, contains $LD_{50}$ or other toxicity data. Unfortunately, many MSDSs contain incomplete and apparently inaccurate information, making them a flawed tool for toxicity assessment. In other countries, labels are quite different, and even less information may be available.

The risk of adverse effects from exposure to household products is difficult to estimate because of the wide variety of products available, the many ingredients they contain, the presence of many "trade secret" ingredients, and the wide variety of exposure scenarios. It is worth noting that the highest exposures to household products are typically to those most likely to be particularly susceptible: children, the elderly, and the chronically ill. These groups tend to spend on average more time in the home than adults aged 20 to 60, who are more likely to work outside the home and to be in good health. Children also exhibit behaviors that increase their exposure to toxic agents in the home: they play on the floor, they put their hands in their mouth, and they are curious about their surroundings. Combined with their low body weight, proportionately higher intake of food and water, and their developmental stage, these behavioral factors contribute to elevated risks.

Risks are undoubtedly increased when products are not used as directed. Examples might include using concentrates at full strength, mixing products with incompatible chemicals, using with inadequate ventilation, or deliberately inhaling solvents to get high. Reasons for "misusing" products are many:

- Label too difficult to read (e.g. too small, not in native language, poorly written).
- Consumer doesn't bother to read label.
- Directions too difficult or inconvenient (what is "adequate" ventilation?).

Nevertheless, even when used as directed, some products may cause significant health risks. Estimates of health risks are often controversial because they involve various assumptions about exposure that are difficult to measure and because the risk assessor may have a financial stake in the outcome. There are many examples of consumer products that have been banned or taken off the market because of unacceptable health or environmental risks: the pesticides chlorpyrifos and diazinon, DDT; the wood preservatives pentachlorophenol and creosote; arsenic-treated lumber; carbon tetrachloride; and lead-based paint. Since the risk of using these products didn't change on the day they were taken off the market, one can infer that the products were unsafe before removal. Given the huge number of consumer products on the market and entering the market every year, regulatory agencies will typically be delayed in identifying unsafe products.

## 18.5 Risk reduction

The risk from using household products can be reduced by reducing the hazard level (toxicity), by reducing exposure, or both. Reducing the toxicity – choosing less-toxic products – is arguably the best strategy because safer product choices can do more than reduce risk in the home. Safer products may also use fewer toxic chemicals in their manufacture and may be safer for the environment when disposed of.

When no safer alternatives are available, reducing exposure becomes especially important. Usually, product labels will explain the recommended safety equipment and procedures appropriate for a particular product. In addition to safety gear, ventilation, and mixing precautions, labels may also mention storage requirements. Unfortunately, some label directions are not specific enough to ensure that following them will guarantee safe use.

Label-directed or common sense precautions should always be taken, even when using products with relatively low toxicity. For example, all chemical products should be kept out of children's reach.

Innovative programs are also available to help home residences reduce exposure to toxic substances. The Master Home Environmentalist program of the American Lung Association trains volunteers to visit homes and conduct a Home Environmental Assessment. Home residences are encouraged to make changes to reduce exposures to toxic substance. A major focus of this program is on reducing asthma in children.

**Table 18.4 Least-toxic alternatives**

| Alternative | Instead of using | Toxic ingredient avoided |
|---|---|---|
| Latex paint | Oil-based paint | Solvents |
| Snake, plunger | Caustic drain opener | Corrosive lye |
| Scouring powder | Acid toilet cleaner | Corrosive hydrochloric acid |
| Beneficial nematodes | Insecticide for soil grubs | Diazinon, carbaryl, or other insecticide |
| Weed puller, mulch | Herbicide | 2,4-D, dichlobenil, etc. |

## 18.6 Safer alternatives

Avoiding the use of toxic products can take the form of avoiding chemical products altogether for certain jobs, choosing products made from safer ingredients, and buying ready-to-use dilutions rather than concentrates. Table 18.4 shows some examples of less-toxic alternatives for common products.

A few additional words are necessary regarding alternatives to pesticides. Pest control is a complex process involving living organisms that can often be difficult to control using a single method. Integrated pest management (IPM) is a decision-making process that utilizes preventative strategies, careful monitoring, realistic pest tolerances, and natural enemies to reduce the need for chemical pesticides. Although chemical pesticides may be used in IPM, a good IPM program typically reduces chemical use considerably and attempts to use those chemicals that will minimize human and environmental impacts. Household pest control can follow the same strategies, using non-chemical methods whenever possible and choosing lower-impact pesticides if chemicals are necessary.

## 18.7 Recommendations

Although the risks of household products are difficult to estimate, taking common-sense precautions can easily reduce them:

- Minimize purchase of toxic or otherwise hazardous products.
- Store all chemical products out of children's reach.
- Read and follow label directions.
- Dispose of hazardous products in accordance with local regulations.

It is difficult for consumers to identify least-toxic products by comparing product labels. Government agencies could do much more to assist and protect consumers:

- Government agencies should require that all product ingredients be listed on product labels. This practice would allow product users to understand product hazards better and to avoid ingredients they are allergic to or don't wish to purchase.

- Government agencies in the United States that regulate product labels should harmonize their labeling systems to avoid inconsistencies between products that are regulated by different agencies.

## 18.8 More information and references

### 18.8.1 Slide presentation

- A Small Dose of Toxics in the Home presentation material. Online. Available HTTP: <http://www.crcpress.com/e_products/> and follow the links to downloads and then the catalog number TF1691.
  Web site contains presentation material related to toxics in the home.

### 18.8.2 European, Asian, and international agencies

- England – Department of Health – Wired for Health. Online. Available HTTP: <http://www.wiredforhealth.gov.uk/> (accessed: 10 April 2003).
  Wired for Health is a wonderful site with information for students, parents, and teachers on healthy homes and schools.
- World Health Organization – Child Health. Online. Available HTTP: <http://www.who.int/health_topics/child_health/en/> (accessed: 10 April 2003).
  Site has information on global child health issues.

### 18.8.3 North American agencies

- US Environmental Protection Agency – Household Waste Management. Online. Available HTTP: <http://www.epa.gov/seahome/hwaste.html> (accessed: 10 April 2003).
  Site has a self-directed educational program on managing household waste.
- US Environmental Protection Agency – Envir $ense. Online. Available HTTP: <http://es.epa.gov/techinfo/facts/safe-fs.html> (accessed: 10 April 2003).
  Site has fact sheet on safe substitutes at home – non-toxic household products.
- US Environmental Protection Agency – Office of Pollution Prevention & Toxics (OPPT). Online. Available HTTP: <http://www.epa.gov/opptintr/> (accessed: 10 April 2003).
  The site promotes safer chemicals and risk education.
- US Environmental Protection Agency – Indoor Air Quality (IAQ). Online. Available HTTP: <http://www.epa.gov/air/indoorair/> (accessed: 10 April 2003).
  This site contains information on indoor air and related health issues.
- California – Office of Environmental Health Hazard Assessment – Education – Art Hazards. Online. Available HTTP: <http://www.oehha.org/education/art/> (accessed: 10 April 2003).
  Site has information on hazardous art supplies and substitutes.

### 18.8.4 Non-government organizations

■ American Lung Association of Washington (ALAW) http://www.alaw.org/> (accessed: 10 April 2003).
Site has information on childhood asthma and the Master Home Environmentalist Program.

■ American Association of Poison Control Centers (AAPCC). Online. Available HTTP: <http://www.aapcc.org/> (accessed: 10 April 2003).
"AAPCC is a nationwide organization of poison centers and interested individuals."

■ California Poison Control System (CPCS). Online. Available HTTP: <http://www.calpoison.org/> (accessed: 10 April 2003).
Site has wide range of information on poisons in and around the home.

■ Non-Toxic.info. Online. Available HTTP: <http://www.non-toxic.info/index.htm> (accessed: 10 April 2003).
This site provides "information about dangerous chemicals found in cosmetics and personal care products, in common cleansers we use at home and at work, and in toxic products we may expose ourselves to every day".

■ Center for Health, Environment and Justice – Child Proofing our Communities Campaign. Online. Available HTTP: <http://www.childproofing.org> (accessed: 10 April 2003).
Site is "geared to protect children from exposures to environmental health hazards."

■ Washington Toxics Coalition (WTC). Online. Available HTTP: <www.watoxics.org> (accessed: 10 April 2003).
WTC provides information on model pesticide policies, alternatives to home pesticides, information on persistent chemical pollutants, and much more.

■ Washington State, Seattle – Environment. Online. Available HTTP: <http://www.cityofseattle.net/environment/> (accessed: 10 April 2003).
Site covers information on encouraging a sustainable environment including purchasing less toxic products.

■ Green Seal. Online. Available HTTP: <http://www.greenseal.org/> (accessed: 10 April 2003).
Green Seal encourages the purchasing of products and services that cause less toxic pollution and waste.

■ Washington State, King County – Household Hazardous Waste. Online. Available HTTP: <http://www.metrokc.gov/hazwaste/house/> (accessed: 10 April 2003).
Site contains information on managing and disposing of household hazardous products and waste.

### 18.8.5 References

■ A Guide to Health Risk Assessment. California Environmental Protection Agency, Office of Environmental Health Hazard Assessment. Available as a pdf file. Online. Available HTTP: <http://www.oehha.org/risk/layperson/index.html> (accessed: 10 April 2003).

■   Litovitz, T. L., Klein-Schwartz, W., White, S., Cobaugh, D., Youniss, J., Omslaer, J., Drab, A. and Benson, B. (2001). Annual Report of the American Association of Poison Control Centers Toxic Exposures Surveillance System. Am. J. Emergency Med, 19(5), 337–396.

■   Ott, W, R. and Roberts, J. (1998). Everyday exposure to toxic pollutants. Scientific American, February.

# Chapter 19

## Risk assessment and risk management

## Contents

- Introduction and history
- Risk assessment
- Risk management
- Precautionary principle
- More information and references

## 19.1 Introduction and history

Risk assessment is both old and new. Old in the sense that humans and animals survive by evaluating the risk of harm verses the benefits of action. For early humans, the hunt for food or eating a new plant involved risk of harm, but doing nothing risked starvation. In our current society, this kind of informal risk assessment is now more directed towards the risks of eating undercooked hamburger or riding a bicycle without a helmet. More formally, risk assessment now refers to a mathematical calculation of risk based on toxicity and exposure.

> If someone had evaluated the risk of fire right after it was invented they may well have decided to eat their food raw.
> Julian Morris of the Institute of Economic Affairs in London

Concern about the risk of chemical exposures also has a long history. For a period of time, food poisons were a concern for those in power.

> What is food to one man may be fierce poison to others.
> Lucretius (c. 99–c. 55 BC)

Percivall Pott made one of the first observations of a health risk related to occupational exposure. In 1775, he noted that chimney sweeps had a higher incidence of cancer of the scrotum. A century later, in 1895, it was observed that workers in the aniline dye industry were more likely to develop bladder cancer.

The number of workers exposed to chemicals grew rapidly with the onset of the industrial revolution and advances in chemical engineering. One of the first efforts to evaluate systematically the risk of exposure to chemicals began in 1938 by a group convened in Washington, DC, that subsequently became the American Conference of Governmental Industrial Hygienists (ACGIH). In 1941 the Chemical Substances Committee was established and charged with investigating and recommending exposure limits for chemical substances. They established exposure limits or threshold limit values (TLVs) for 148 chemicals. ACGIH now publishes a list of TLVs for 642 chemical substances and physical agents and 38 biological exposure indices for selected chemicals.

In 1958, in response to the increased awareness that chemicals can cause cancer, the US Congress passed the Delaney clause, which prohibited the addition to the food supply of any substance known to cause cancer in animals or humans. Compared with today's standards, the analytical methods to detect a potentially harmful substance were very poor. As the analytical methods improved, it became apparent that the food supply had low levels of substances that were known to cause cancer in either animals or humans. The obvious question was: Is a small amount of a substance "safe" to consume. This question in turn raised many others about how to interpret data or extrapolate data to very low doses. The 1970s saw a flourishing of activity to develop and refine risk assessment methodologies.

The initial focus was to develop risk assessment procedures to establish exposure limits for cancer-causing substances, the primary concerns being the food supply and the workplace. These efforts were gradually expanded to include non-cancer endpoints such as nervous system development, reproductive effects, and effects on the immune system. Researchers at national and international agencies are developing better approaches to dealing with uncertainty in health effects data and the resulting need to apply judgment in interpreting the results. The area of judgment is a critical aspect of risk assessment. The process of interpreting and communicating risk assessment results requires full understanding and disclosure of the assumptions, data gaps, and possible financial interests that may play a role. Concerned by the shortcomings of risk assessment, a growing body of scientists is advocating a precautionary approach to risks that are not fully understood. The precautionary principle has been applied to issues related to toxicology, public health, and sustainable development and use of the environment (Cairns, 2003; Goldstein, 2001) and is an established global principle (Rio Declaration, 1992).

In order to protect the environment, the precautionary approach shall be widely applied by States according to their capabilities. Where there are threats of serious or irreversible damage, lack of full scientific certainty shall not be used as a reason for postponing cost-effective measures to prevent environmental degradation.

Principle 15: Rio Declaration 1992

## 19.2 Risk assessment

# Hazard × exposure = risk

Risk assessment is a multi-step process to relate the association of exposure to a chemical or physical agent with adverse outcome. Initially the focus was human health but now it has broadened to include wider environmental and ecological concerns. Risk management is a more overtly political process directed at determining an action based on relevant public and environmental health goals, cost, societal issues, and other related or even unrelated issues. An important part of risk management is balancing the risks, costs, and benefits – never an easy task.

---

Risk assessment is the process of estimating association between an exposure to a chemical or physical agent and the incidence of some adverse outcome.

**Steps in risk assessment**

- Hazard identification
- Exposure assessment
- Dose–response assessment
- Risk characterization

---

The first step in risk assessment is to gather health-related information associated with an exposure. Ideally, hazard identification starts before there is significant use of the agent. The structure of the compound is compared with that of compounds with known toxicity profiles. Cell-based studies are often performed to screen for toxicity. Finally, animal bioassays and human studies are performed to characterize and develop a toxicity profile. Multiple health-related endpoints are evaluated to determine if the compound is associated with adverse effects. Advantages of animal studies include experimental control and accurate knowledge of the dose.

Using knowledge gained from animal studies or observations from human populations, a more formal human epidemiology study may be performed. Human studies have the obvious advantage of being done on the subject of most interest, but they are time consuming and expensive, and often have many variables that are difficult to control.

---

**Common toxicity endpoints for hazard identification**

- Carcinogenicity
- Mutations
- Altered immune function

- Teratogenicity
- Altered reproductive function
- Neurobehavioral toxicity
- Organ-specific effects
- Ecological effects (wildlife, environmental persistence)

If the hazard assessment indicates that the compound is potentially hazardous, the next step is to evaluate the various possibilities for exposure. What is the most likely route of exposure: oral, inhalation or skin? How much absorption is expected from the different routes of exposure? Information is also needed on amount, duration, and frequency of exposure. Is exposure occurring in the home, workplace, school, or other areas? This information helps to define the population of concern. Exposure information may also be important for designing appropriate studies on hazard assessment and certainly for the next step of establishing dose–response relationships.

**Exposure assessment**

- Route of exposure (skin, oral, inhalation)
- Amount of exposure (dose)
- Duration and frequency of exposure
- To whom (animals, humans, environment)

Next, it is important to characterize the dose–response relationship for the agent. Data from the initial hazard assessment, combined with exposure assessment information, are used to determine the most sensitive endpoint. Available data are used to define the dose at which there is no observed effect (NOAEL – no observed adverse effect level) and the shape of the dose–response curve (Figure 19.1). It may be necessary to perform additional studies to define the dose–response curve.

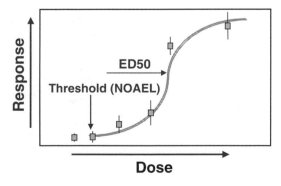

**Figure 19.1.** Dose–response curve.

The final step is to take all the information from hazard assessment, exposure assessment, and dose–response assessment and summarize it in a risk characterization for the chemical substance. Any uncertainties in the data set or missing information must be evaluated. While all efforts are made to minimize professional judgment by having robust data, it is often the case that not enough of the right information is available. Recommendations must still be made as to an acceptable level of exposure for a given population, the goal being to ensure the even the most sensitive individuals are protected from any adverse effects. The dose thought to ensure protection is called a reference dose (RfD) or acceptable daily intake (ADI). Note the word safe is NOT used, only the avoidance of adverse effects.

Acceptable daily intake (ADI)

The daily intake of chemical, which during an entire lifetime appears to be without appreciable risk on the basis of all known facts at the time.

WHO (1962)

There are of course many mathematically complex ways to perform a risk assessment, but first key questions about the biological data must be resolved. The most sensitive endpoint must be defined along with relevant toxicity and dose–response data. A standard risk assessment approach that is often used is the so-called "divide by 10 rule". Dividing the dose by 10 applies a safety factor to ensure that even the most sensitive individuals are protected. Animal studies are typically used to establish a dose–response curve and the most sensitive endpoint. From the dose–response curve a NOAEL dose or no observed adverse effect level is derived. This is the dose at which there appears to be no adverse effects in the animal studies at a particular endpoint, which could be cancer, liver damage, or a neurobehavioral effect. This dose is then divided by 10 if the animal data are in any way thought to be inadequate. For example, there may be a great deal of variability, or there were adverse effects at the lowest dose, or there were only tests of short-term exposure to the chemical. An additional factor of 10 is used when extrapolating from animals to humans. Last, a factor of 10 is used to account for variability in the human population or to account for sensitive individuals such as children or the elderly. The final number is the reference dose (RfD) or acceptable daily intake (ADI). This process is summarized below.

Safety factors are typically used in a risk assessment to define an acceptable dose for food additives and pesticides. It is obviously very important to ensure that an artificial sweetener such as aspartame, which is commonly used in artificially sweetened drinks, has a large margin of safety. All age groups, as well as pregnant women, consume artificial sweeteners, so they must have a large margin of safety. Some factors to consider are given in Table 19.1.

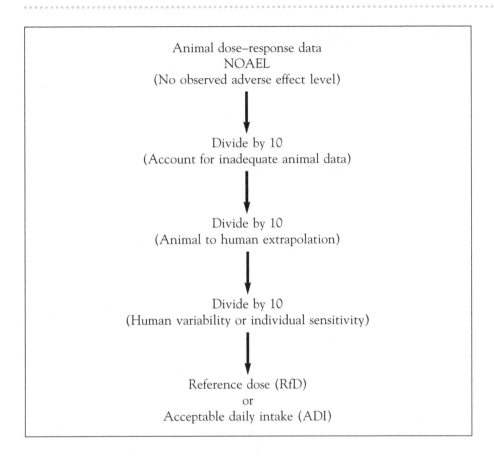

Animal dose–response data
NOAEL
(No observed adverse effect level)

↓

Divide by 10
(Account for inadequate animal data)

↓

Divide by 10
(Animal to human extrapolation)

↓

Divide by 10
(Human variability or individual sensitivity)

↓

Reference dose (RfD)
or
Acceptable daily intake (ADI)

---

**Table 19.1 Factors to consider**

| Route of exposure | |
|---|---|
| Ingestion | Concentration of toxicant in ingested material, amount consumed, frequency of ingestion, absorption factor |
| Skin | Concentration of toxicant in applied material, skin area exposed, absorption factor |
| Inhalation | Concentration of toxicant in air, breathing rate, exposure time, absorption factor |

## 19.3 Risk management

Risk management is the process of deciding what to do to reduce a known or suspected risk. Risk management balances the various community demands with the scientific information generated from the risk assessment. Public perception of risk is also considered. Table 19.2 characterizes some of the factors that influence perception of risk. An individual's perception of risk is sometimes very different from a risk

**Table 19.2 Characteristics of risk**

| Characteristic | Level | Examples |
|---|---|---|
| Knowledge | Little known | Food additives |
| | Much known | Alcoholic drinks |
| Newness | Old | Guns |
| | New | Space travel |
| Voluntariness | Not voluntary | Crime |
| | Voluntary | Rock climbing |
| Control | Not controllable | Natural disasters |
| | Controllable | Smoking |
| Dreadedness | Little dread | Vaccination |
| | Great dread | Nerve gas |
| Catastrophic potential | Not likely | Sunbathing |
| | Likely | War |
| Equity | Distributed | Skiing |
| | Undistributed | Hazardous dump |

Adapted from Kraus and Slovic (1988).

assessment from a more objective analysis of the data. For example, individuals often rank nuclear power as a high risk but most experts give it a low risk rank.

Early risk evaluation often just looked at death as the main endpoint, asking if a particular action or exposure led to increases in death or reduced number of working years. Advances in the biological sciences have required that more complex risk analysis be undertaken to evaluate quality of life issues and not just death as an endpoint. The challenge for both risk assessment and risk management will be to take into consideration quality of life and individual values into the decision-making process.

## 19.4 Precautionary principle

When an activity raises threats of harm to the environment or human health, precautionary measures should be taken even if some cause and effect relationships are not fully established scientifically.

Wingspread Statement on the Precautionary Principle, Jan. 1998.

Another approach to risk-based decision-making is the precautionary principle. The risk assessment and risk management approach used in the United States places a heavy reliance on the certainty of the data. The precautionary principle emphasizes that there is always some uncertainty and that decisions should be based on recognizing the possibility of harm. When in doubt, be cautious until adequate data are available to show that there is little potential for harm. Action to reduce exposure to hazardous agents should begin even if there is some uncertainty in the data.

In other words, some uncertainty in the data should not be used as an excuse for inaction. This approach is being given more consideration in Europe than in the United States. The approach gains credibility when one considers how its application years ago would have prevented the tragic effects of lead in gasoline and paint.

## 19.5 More information and references

### 19.5.1 Slide presentation

- A Small Dose of Risk Assessment presentation material. Online. Available HTTP: <http://www.crcpress.com/e_products/> and follow the links to downloads and then the catalog number TF1691.
  Web site contains presentation material related to risk assessment.

### 19.5.2 European, Asian, and international agencies

- England – Department of Health – Risk Research. Online. Available HTTP: <http://www.doh.gov.uk/risk/index.htm> (accessed: 10 April 2003).
  The Department of Health has published information and research outcomes on risk and public health.
- World Health Organization – The International Programme on Chemical Safety (IPCS) – Risk Assessment. Online. Available HTTP: <http://www.who.int/pcs/ra_main.html> (accessed: 10 April 2003).
  Information on global risk assessment issues.
- EnviroLink – The Online Environmental Community. Online. Available HTTP: <http://www.envirolink.org/> (accessed: 10 April 2003).
  "EnviroLink is a non-profit organization . . . a grassroots online community that unites hundreds of organizations and volunteers around the world with millions of people in more than 150 countries. EnviroLink is dedicated to providing comprehensive, up-to-date environmental information and news."

### 19.5.3 North American agencies

- US Environmental Protection Agencies – National Center for Environmental Assessment (NCEA). Online. Available HTTP: <http://cfpub.epa.gov/ncea/> (accessed: 10 April 2003).
  NCEA goals are to apply "science to improve risk assessment and environmental decision making."
- California Office of Environmental Health Hazard Assessment (OEHHA). Risk Assessment – Online. Available HTTP: <http://www.oehha.org/risk.html> (accessed: 10 April 2003).
  "OEHHA is responsible for developing and providing risk managers in state and local government agencies with toxicological and medical information relevant to decisions involving public health."
- US Brookhaven National Laboratory – Safety & Health Services Chemical Management. Online. Available HTTP: <http://www.bnl.gov/esh/shsd/cms/Safety_Carcinogens.htm> (accessed: 10 April 2003).

Site contains a comprehensive table listing chemicals and compares their designation as carcinogens by national and international agencies.

### 19.5.4 Non-government organizations

- American Conference of Governmental Industrial Hygienists (ACGIH). Online. Available HTTP: <http://www.acgih.org/> (accessed: 10 April 2003). "The ACGIS community of professionals advances worker health and safety through education and the development and dissemination of scientific and technical knowledge.

- Toxicology Excellence for Risk Assessment (TERA). Online. Available HTTP: <http://www.tera.org/> (accessed: 10 April 2003). "TERA is a nonprofit[501(c)(3)] corporation dedicated to the best use of toxicity data for the development of risk values."

- Society for Risk Analysis (SRA). Online. Available HTTP: <http://www.sra.org/> (accessed: 10 April 2003). "SRA provides an open forum for all those who are interested in risk analysis. Risk analysis is broadly defined to include risk assessment, risk characterization, risk communication, risk management, and policy relating to risk."

- Harvard Center for Risk Analysis. Online. Available HTTP: <http://www.hcra.harvard.edu/> (accessed: 10 April 2003). This Center focuses on "using decision science to empower informed choices about risks to health, safety, and the environment."

- The Hampshire Research Institute (HRI). Online. Available HTTP: <http://www.hampshire.org/> (accessed: 10 April 2003). "HRI uses scientific, engineering, and computing expertise to make a difference on environmental issues."

- Ag BioTech InfoNet – Precautionary Principle. Online. Available HTTP: <http://www.biotech-info.net/precautionary.html> (accessed: 10 April 2003). Site has wide array information on the precautionary principle.

- The Science & Environmental Health Network – Precautionary Principle. Online. Available HTTP: <http://www.sehn.org/precaution.html> (accessed: 10 April 2003). SEHN advocates the wise application of science to protecting the environment and public health.

### 19.5.5 References

- A Guide to Health Risk Assessment. California Environmental Protection Agency, Office of Environmental Health Hazard Assessment. Available as a pdf file. Online. Available HTTP: <http://www.oehha.org/risk/layperson/index.html> (accessed: 10 April 2003).

- The Precautionary Principle In Action, a Handbook. Science and Environmental Health Network, Joel Tickner, Carolyn Raffensperger, and Nancy Myers. Online. Available HTTP: <http://www.biotech-info.net/precautionary.html> (accessed: 10 April 2003).

- Cairns, J., Jr. (2003). Interrelationships between the Precautionary Principle, Prediction Strategies, and Sustainable Use of the Planet. Environmental Health Perspectives Volume 111, Number 7, June 2003.
- Goldstein, B. D. (2001). The precautionary principle and public health – the precautionary principle also applies to public health actions. Am. J. Public Health, 91(9), 1358–1361.
- Kraus, N. N. and Slovic, P. (1988). Risk Analysis, 8(3): 435–455.
- Rio Declaration on Environment and Development. Stockholm, Sweden: United Nations; 1992. Publication E. 73.II.A.14. Online. Available HTTP: <http://www.un.org/documents/ga/conf151/aconf15126-1annex1.htm> (accessed: 6 July 2003).
- WHO (1962). Principles in governing consumer safety in relation to pesticide residues. WHO Tech Rep Ser, 240.

# Glossary

| Term | Definition | Example |
|------|-----------|---------|
| Absorption | The process by which an agent is taken into the blood supply or cells of an organism. | Absorption of nicotine by the lungs |
| Acute exposure | A singe or very limited number of doses | One alcoholic drink |
| Acute response | The response associated with acute exposure | Drunk from an evening drinking alcohol |
| Acute toxicity | Undesirable effects of an acute exposure | Hangover from alcohol |
| ADI | Acceptable daily intake – "The daily intake of chemical, which during an entire lifetime appears to be without appreciable risk on the basis of all known facts at that time" | Food additives, pesticides |
| Anemia | Decreased ability of blood to transport oxygen | Fewer or damaged red blood cells (lead) |
| Asbestosis | A progressive, non-cancerous disease causing shortness of breath from scarring of the lung due to asbestos exposure | Asbestos workers |
| Bioaccumulate | The ability of some organisms to accumulate specific compounds | Fish accumulate methyl mercury; DDT or PCBs accumulate in fat |
| Biotransformation | An organism changing one substance into another form often to increase excretion or reduce toxicity | Bacteria changing mercury into methyl mercury |

| Term | Definition | Example |
|------|------------|---------|
| Carcinogen or carcinogenic | Any substance that causes cancer | Asbestos |
| Chelating agent | An agent that binds other agents to facilitate their excretion | Used to treat elevated lead or mercury levels |
| Chromosome | Parts of cells responsible for heredity characteristics – DNA | Most humans have 46 chromosomes |
| Chronic toxicity | Causes health effects from long-term exposure | Smoking cigarettes |
| Corrosive | Causes burns to the skin or other body tissue | Lye, strong cleaning agents |
| Detoxification or biotransformation | The biochemical process to neutralize a toxicant (i.e. metabolism) or excretion | The metabolism of alcohol |
| Distribution | How a chemical agent distributes throughout the body | PCBs and pesticides accumulate in fat |
| Dose | A measured amount of exposure – usually in terms of body weight or sometimes surface area | 10 mg/kg |
| Dose–response | The effect or response is related to the dose or amount of exposure to an agent | One cup of coffee is fine but two or three result in unpleasant effects |
| Erythema | Sunburn – inflammation – dilation of the blood vessels thus the redness and heat | UV radiation |
| Excretion | How the body removes agents from the body or even cells | Mercury is excreted in the urine |
| Exposure | Duration and type of contact with an agent | |
| • Route of exposure | How the agent gained access to the organism – dermal (skin), inhalation (lung), stomach (ingestion) | Cigarette smoke – lung Lead – ingestion |
| • Frequency of exposure | How often the exposure occurs and the time between exposures | Consider 4 beers in 1 hour vs 4 beers over 4 days |
| • Duration | How long the exposure occurs – (see acute and chronic exposure) | Acute exposure to gas fumes at a gas station or lifetime exposure to food additives |
| Fetal alcohol syndrome (FAS) | Pattern of physical, developmental, and nervous system disabilities seen in babies born to mothers who consumed alcohol during pregnancy . . . | 1 to 3 per 1000 infants affected worldwide |

| Term | Definition | Example |
|---|---|---|
| Fetal alcohol effect (FAE) | Similar to FAS with learning and nervous system disabilities without the obvious physical deformities | Incidence unknown |
| Half-life | A measure of time to reduce the amount of agent by one-half | The half-life of caffeine in the blood is 3–4 hours |
| Hazard | An agent or situation capable of causing an adverse effect or harm | Loud noise – deafness Lead – reduced IQ |
| Inhalation | Exposure to and absorption of a compound via the lungs | Cigarettes (nicotine) Marijuann (THC) |
| Ingestion | Exposure to and absorption of a compound via the stomach or intestines | Food, coffee (caffeine), lead |
| $LD_{50}$ | Lethal dose that will kill 50% of a group of animals | Ethyl alcohol (10 000 mg/kg) Nicotine (1 mg/kg) |
| Leukemia | Cancer of the blood-forming organs of the bone marrow | Caused by benzene |
| Mesothelioma | A rare cancer of the thin membranes lining the lungs almost always related to asbestos exposure | Asbestos workers (increased with smoking) |
| Metabolism | Change one substance into another, which usually aids excretion or reduces toxicity | Caffeine into less active compounds |
| Milligram (mg) | One thousandth of a gram | 1 mg |
| Minimal risk levels (MRLs) | ATSDR definition – "An MRL is an estimate of the daily human exposure to a hazardous substance that is likely to be without appreciable risk of adverse noncancer health effects over a specified duration of exposure." | Inorganic mercury in air – inhalation 0.2 $\mu g/m^3$ |
| Mutagen or mutagenic | Any substance that causes alterations in cellular DNA | Many cancer-causing agents, radiation |
| Neurotoxicity | Produces an adverse change in the structure or function of the nervous system following exposure to a chemical or physical agent | Mercury, lead, pesticides, heroin, alcohol etc. |
| Neurotransmitter | A chemical used to communicate between cells of the nervous system | Dopamine, serotonin |
| NOAEL | No observed adverse effect level | Dose in mg/kg |
| PCBs | Polychlorinated biphenyls – used as cooling agent in transformers because of low flammability. Now banned because of their environmental persistence and bioaccumulation in fat of many species including whales and humans | Memory loss |

| Term | Definition | Example |
|---|---|---|
| Pesticide | ". . . any substance or mixture of substances intended for preventing, destroying, repelling or mitigating any insects, rodents, nematodes, fungi, or weeds or any other form of life declared to be pests. . . . and any substance or mixture of substances intended for use as a plant regulator, defoliant or desiccant."<br>Federal Insecticide, Fungicide, and Rodenticide Act (FIFRA – 1947) | DDT |
| Pharmacology | The study of the beneficial and adverse effects of drugs | Benefits of aspirin or caffeine |
| Pollutant | An agent, often released by human activity, that is adversely affecting the environment | DDT, PCBs, mercury, lead, etc. |
| Reference dose (RfD) | A daily exposure level (dose) that is not expected to cause any adverse health effects in humans | EPA RfD for methyl mercury – 0.1 µg/kg per day |
| Response | The reaction to an exposure to or dose of an agent | Stomach ache from eating too many green apples |
| Risk | The probability of injury, disease, loss of function, or death for an individual or population exposed to a hazardous substance (risk = hazard × exposure) | Evaluating the dose of lead or mercury that causes developmental effects in children |
| Risk assessment | The process by which the nature and magnitude of risks are identified | Reference dose (RfD) or acceptable daily intake (ADI) |
| Risk communication | Strategies for effectively communicating information about hazards and risk | Town meetings, pamphlets, the World Wide Web |
| Risk management | The process of determining whether or how much to reduce risk through our actions | Hazardous waste site clean up |
| Skin absorption | Exposure to and absorption of a compound via the skin | Nicotine patch, solvents |
| Susceptibility | Factors that can increase or decrease the adverse effects of an agent | Developing organism, childhood, genetics |
| • Age | The young and elderly are often more susceptible to the effects of an agent | Lead is far more toxic to infants than adults |
| • Gender | Men and women differ in their response to agents owing to hormonal influences | Female birth control pill is the most obvious |
| • Health | Disease can increase susceptibility to an agent | Liver disease can increase susceptibility |

| Term | Definition | Example |
|------|-----------|---------|
| • Pregnancy | The many physiological changes that occur during pregnancy alter susceptibility | Greater absorption of lead, longer half-life of caffeine |
| Teratogen or teratogenic | Any substance that causes defects in the developing embryo or fetus (birth defects) | Alcohol can cause facial deformities (FAS) |
| Teratology | From the Greek word *teras* meaning abnormal form, the branch of science that deals with the causes, mechanisms, manifestations and prevention of congenital defects | Thalidomide (caused limb deformities in children) |
| Therapeutic index | Measure of a drug's benefit and safety. A wide index indicates that a drug has few toxic effects at high levels | Wide index – antibiotics Narrow index – lithium |
| Toxic substance (regulatory term) | Any substance that can cause acute or chronic injury to the human body or is suspected to do so | US NIOSH publishes a list of toxic substances |
| Toxicant (poison) | An agent cable of causing toxicity – a poison | DDT, lead, noise, solvents, food additives, ozone |
| Toxicity or toxic effect | An adverse reaction of the organism | Soft egg shells, reduced IQ, cancer |
| Toxicokinetics or pharmacokinetics | The study of absorption, distribution and excretion of an agent | How long alcohol stays in the body |
| Toxicology | The study of the adverse effects of chemical and physical agents on living organisms | Study of affects of lead on the developing nervous system |
| Toxicologist | A scientist who studies the adverse effects of agents on biological systems | |
| Toxin | A natural biological agent (from plants, animals, bacteria, or fungi) that causes toxicity | Domoic acid found in shellfish, caffeine |
| Xenobiotic | A foreign compound, i.e. one that is not naturally found in an organism | Caffeine in humans |

# Abbreviations

## Units of measure

| Abbreviation | Definition |
| --- | --- |
| μg | Microgram (0.000001 gram, one millionth of a gram) |
| mg | Milligram (0.001 grams, one thousandth of a gram) |
| kg | Kilogram (1000 grams, 2.2 lbs) |
| ml | Milliliter (0.001 liter, one thousandth of a liter) |
| dl | One tenth of a liter (100 ml) |
| l | Liter (1.056 liquid quart) |
| lbs | Pounds (0.45 kg) |
| oz | Ounce (28 grams) |

## US Government agencies

| Abbreviation | Definition |
| --- | --- |
| ACGIH | American Conference of Governmental Industrial Hygienists |
| ATSDR | Agency for Toxic Substances and Disease Registry |
| CDC | Centers for Disease Control |
| EPA | Environmental Protection Agency |
| FDA | Food and Drug Administration |
| NIOSH | National Institute for Occupational Safety and Health |
| OSHA | Occupational Safety & Health Administration |
| USGS | US Geological Survey |

# Appendix – Demonstration of the principles of dose-response

- Definitions:
  *Dose* is the amount of exposure to an agent.
  Response is the reaction to the dose.
  For example, eating one green apple may be just fine but eating five green apples at one time may produce a very undesirable response.
- Materials required:
  Four large size glasses (wine glasses work very well)
  One small size glass
  Food color (blue is best, in container to dispense drops)
  One pitcher of water

### Demonstration of the importance of amount of the dose (see Figure A1)

Fill three large glasses with approximately ³/₄ water. This represents the approximate water content of an individual. I usually ask the class how much water is in each of them – makes for a fun discussion.

Put one drop of blue food color in the first glass, three in the second glass, and then six to nine in the last glass. Ask the class to count with you and how many they would like to have in the last glass.

Stir with a pencil or pen and discuss the change in color as a response to increased dose of food color in each glass. Discuss how some chemicals, caffeine being one, distribute throughout total body water.

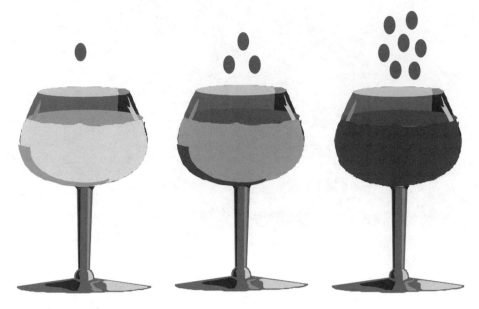

The Greater the Dose, The Greater the Effect

**Figure A1.** Effects of amount on response.

### Demonstration of the importance of size (see Figure A2)

Fill one large glass and the small glass with approximately $^3/_4$ water. The small glass represents a small child in contrast to the adult-size glass.

Put one drop of food color in each glass. The small glass will be much darker and usually look like the high-dose glass from the first demonstration.

Discuss the importance of size and the impact weight has on dose, depending on sophistication of the group. A small child who consumes one can of caffeinated drink will have a very different response from an adult because of the difference in the dose of caffeine relative to body size.

For exposure to a chemical agent, dose is usually expressed in relation to body weight. This is because for a fixed amount of toxic agent, the dose, and likewise the effect, depends directly on weight. We know, for example, that one shot of alcohol would have a very big effect on a child weighting 10 lbs and a much smaller effect on an adult weighing 200 lbs. To take this into account, dose is measured in units of milligrams of toxicant per kilogram of body weight, abbreviated mg/kg. If someone consumed 100 mg of caffeine, approximately the amount in a cup of coffee or two cans of caffeinated drink, and if they weighed 70 kg (about 155 lbs), the dose would be 100 mg per 70 kg of body weight or 1.4 mg/kg. On the other hand, if a child weighing only 10 kg (about 22 lbs) consumed the same 100 mg of caffeine, the dose would 10 mg/kg, seven times as large because the body weight is one-seventh. Thus size and amount of exposure determine the dose and are critical factors in

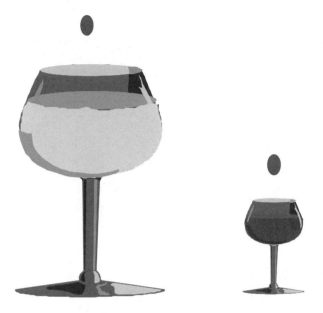

The Smaller the Size, The Greater the Effect

**Figure A2.** Effects of size on response.

toxicology. This principle can be an extremely important factor in home lead or pesticide exposures, where the dose a child receives is far greater than the adult due to the small size and extra sensitivity of the child.

# Index

Boldface page numbers denote the location of the main body of information on the subject.